WALL
STREET
YOGA

BY GURUNANDA
ENTREPRENEUR TURNED YOGI

Healthland LLC
602 N. Canon Drive
Beverly Hills, CA 90210
www.healthlandllc.com

Written by Puneet Nanda
Illustrated by Marguerite Masing
Designed by Kara Kenna

www.gurunanda.com

ISBN: 978-0-9861384-0-9
Printed in the USA

10 9 8 7 6 5 4 3 2 1

GURUNANDA'S HAPPY BREATH YOGA:
WALL STREET YOGA

TABLE OF CONTENTS

FOREWORD

Welcome to **GURUNANDA'S HAPPY BREATH YOGA**. This book is one in a series that I hope will help you incorporate yoga and yogic breathing into your life - simply, quickly and easily. Today, we're all so busy. Stress has become not only common, it's expected. With my Happy Breath Yoga, the only thing you need to know how to do is *breathe*! Sure, I will give you some exercises, tools, tips and guidance, but you are already perfectly equipped to experience more joy, calmness and overall health. In fact, you deserve it!

GURUNANDA'S HAPPY BREATH YOGA goes beyond just books. It's a way of life. It's a way of life that changed *my* life.

ENJOY. LAUGH. MOVE. BREATHE.

- Puneet Nanda
  GuruNanda

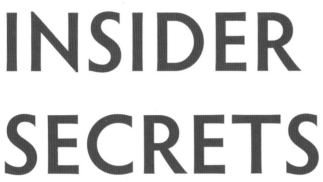

INSIDER
SECRETS

Who in the World is GuruNanda?

"The smart ones are those who learn from others' mistakes instead of suffering themselves."

- GuruNanda

I WAS HERE.

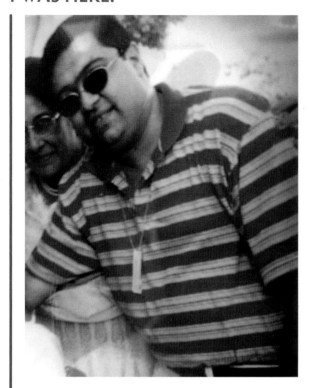
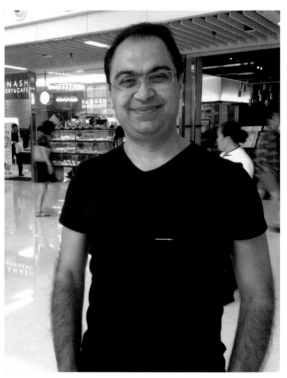

NOW, I'M HERE.

In between, I almost killed myself. I'm not too humble to boast that I was a successful entrepreneur with a multi-million dollar oral care company that strongly competed with the "big guys." I had more than 100 employees, was working 16-hour days and did business across three time zones. I was living the dream. Then, in 2008, I collapsed and was rushed to the hospital with chest pains. After a battery of tests, the doctors informed me that I did not have a heart attack. I had a nervous breakdown.

But let me back up to the "living the dream" part. I grew up in New Delhi, India, where my father ran a small toothbrush company. In college there, I studied medicine because I have always been fascinated by science and the human body - especially how the body works and heals itself. In 1989, my father suffered a heart attack and could no longer run the company, so I took over. I renamed the company Dr. Fresh, a nickname my classmates had cheekily given me at one time for dating the university dean's daughter. My company's inexpensive toothbrushes virtually flew out of the factory and eventually found their way to Russia where free traders were looking for inexpensive consumer products to sell. In 1993, I moved to Moscow to open an office. I was young, fearless and full of energy. However, my exponentially growing business didn't make others there - namely the Russian mafia - as happy as it made me. I was threatened with bodily harm and forced to dip into my rising revenues to pay bosses. Ultimately, my efforts weren't enough and I reached a low point when I was pistol-whipped by thugs until I lost consciousness (I've still got the scars to prove it). After three years in Moscow, I returned to New Delhi with my tail between my legs.

But I knew there was still something more out there, so I set my sights on the United States. Naturally, my closely-knit family was divided about any more adventures for me. I took yet another chance in 1998 and moved to New York, where I soon discovered that trying to sell toothbrushes in the cold of winter was as oppressive as the New Delhi smog. That Christmas, miserable, alone and with a raging fever, I slipped and fell in the snow on the way to the pharmacy. Lying on the ground, I knew I had to find sun. I bought a ticket for Miami and went to the airport, where my flight was promptly cancelled.

Stuck at the airport, I asked a random stranger, "Where can I go where it's sunny 24/7?" "Los Angeles," was the man's answer. I slept the entire flight west and got off that plane to find sun that lasted all day... and days to come. The City of Angels became home for me. I soon sent for my wife and young children, who both loved L.A. as well. There, I scored my first big U.S. deal, selling 180,000 toothbrush six-packs to 99 Cents Only Stores. I was persistent to the point of annoying, but I was filled with passion and creativity. Soon after, I developed a toothbrush that lit up and glowed as a way to get kids to brush longer.

And the rest is history - *my* history, filled with antidepressants and mood stabilizers, tranquilizers for stress, beta blockers, painkillers, Depakote and Lipitor. I was single-handedly keeping the pharmaceutical industry in business.

My weight ballooned from 146 to 186 pounds. I would start my day with phone calls to New York and London while eating a huge omelet with toast and butter, plus cereal and milk. After all, breakfast is the most important meal of the day, right? Not the way *I* was eating it. I'd get to the office to fight ten fires - bills, legal dramas, accounts that wouldn't pay, truck drivers I paid *too* much, and fights among employees. All this chaos only made me hungrier. By mid-morning, I would have a high-calorie, high-sugar "snack bar" and a giant cup of coffee, which didn't quell my constant yawns. When lunchtime arrived, I would drive to the nearest fast food restaurant, order a chicken sandwich, and fool myself into thinking it was healthier than a burger and fries (it's not). I would eat in my car with my Bluetooth in my ear, talking away.

Life seemed boring if I wasn't doing two things at once. Sound familiar?

I would come home at night to a wife who was upset that I had no time for her. My kids were scared to talk to me because they felt they'd be a disturbance. Any problem just seemed to create more chaos and stress, which made me want to stay away from my family and friends, even though I felt so lonely inside.

At night, sitting on the couch watching television, I would usually eat a traditional Indian dinner, which always included too much naan (flatbread) or roti bread. I didn't have the energy to go for a walk or exercise. At bedtime, I would drag myself to the bathroom to brush, then crash, only to wake up three hours later to compulsively plan my next move and fret for another hour or two. By morning, I'd be on my phone call to New York or London... and the cycle started all over again.

Until it didn't... when I almost died.

I ended up in the hospital (read Chapter 9 to find out why). There, a friend of mine... posed this question to me: "Do you know the name of the president of Lebanon?" I didn't. He continued, "That man has spent his entire life devoted to that whole country, and you don't know him. Who the hell knows *you*?" At that moment, my eyes opened. Sure, I was in the Young Presidents Organization (YPO) and was Ernst & Young's Entrepreneur of the Year for 2011. But really, I was just toiling away, day in and day out, with nothing to show for my work except physical illness and emotional heartache. I had to change my life - for myself and *my* family.

I was introduced to an acupuncturist whose assistant nurse suggested yoga's simple Cat-Cow Pose. She assumed that because I was Indian, I was familiar with yoga, but I had forgotten the practice. As I did the basic move, memories flooded back to a yoga class in my elementary school. Back then, I loved the feeling of yoga, but the teacher was scary. In the scorching New Delhi summer heat, he put us through an impossible regimen of poses and would even hit us on the bottom with a stick if we did the moves wrong. My love for yoga was soon replaced by fear. But I remembered how good it felt when we practiced simple deep breaths, raising our hands up and down to clear our minds. The "Om" chanting made me feel free. At that acupuncturist's office, my love for yoga was reawakened.

I realized that I had become a functioning drug addict and wanted to get off of all the pharmaceuticals, especially the tranquilizers. But my first afternoon without them prompted an aching craving. My doctor recommended meditation. At that point, I had no other choice than to give it a go.

At my first meditation retreat at a center run by Deepak Chopra, I met many like-minded people going through the same life changes I was facing. However, the yoga I learned was erratic with no theme - and the practice was optional. **I needed a way of life.** I then learned about Transcendental Meditation (TM), a mantra-based meditation program. But again, I ended up feeling unsatisfied.

It was time to return to India, the birthplace of yoga and meditation. At the advice of my mother, I found myself doing yoga on the banks of the River Ganges, the holiest of all rivers. In mythology, the River Ganges takes in all the ills and sins of everyone who comes to have a dip, and cleanses these toxins away. Each second you're there, you can feel the powerful vortex around you. I discovered an ashram and a teacher who was the most learned and dedicated soul on earth. She taught me simple yoga and inspired me to dedicate my time and energy to simply breathing.

It was so basic:

I NEEDED TO BREATHE.

When I finished my initial regimen at the ashram, I had my first real "Ah-ha!" Moment. I felt stress-free for the first time in decades. I stayed there for the next ten days until I knew I could perform that kind of yoga on my own. After the experience, all I wanted to do was share. So, I sold the company.

As a full-time yoga student, I became dedicated to expanding my knowledge. I read books, attended seminars and traveled the world to deepen my practice and meditation. I used my passion for medical studies to research the science behind each yoga pose and how the moves benefit our bodies. I went to the famous OSHO ashram, the Jindal NatureCure Institute, and several places in Bangalore, Kerala and Pune. I opened my mind to various yogic schools of thought, such as Iyengar, Krishnamacharya and Baba Ramdev. I attended international yoga festivals at Parmarth ashram in Rishikesh, in Bali, Costa Rica and Hawaii. I eventually became an accredited yoga instructor officially affiliated with the Yoga Alliance. I've taught non-profit courses around the world while speaking and lecturing on the power of yogic breathing.

Who gave me the moniker "GuruNanda?" I did. Does it seem pompous to call myself a guru? It's truly not. My favorite teacher suggested it, because the word **"guru" simply means "teacher" in Sanskrit.** A guru is the dispeller of darkness, illuminating the light that's already in all of us. The term is based on the interplay between darkness and light, and I have known both. Unfortunately, "gurus" are now often compared to megalomaniac personalities or "crunchy-granola" caricatures in movies or on TV. I am neither.

And although my oral care brand was called Dr. Fresh, I am not a doctor. I am medical school-trained, with a very strong and extensive science background. But this book and all my recommendations are just one man's opinion. **As with any exercise, fitness or diet program, please consult your doctor first.**

So why should you listen to me?

I am the epitome of the person who needed this book, *Wall Street Yoga*, a Type A personality who couldn't quiet my mind long enough to meditate for even one minute. Trendy "power yoga," with women in sexy, stretchy pants, was overwhelmingly intimidating. Hot yoga made me feel sick and ashamed I couldn't bend my inflexible body into a pretzel. My awakening came when I realized that just being in a pose and deep breathing several times made me feel connected to myself like never before. Sure, yoga is good exercise. In one year, I lost 40 pounds doing it, combined with regular trips to the gym and healthy eating. But yoga is a way of life that *fits into your life.*

Yoga doesn't require a lot of time when you are doing it with a conscious effort to **turn distress into de-stress.**

Breath is a direct bridge between body and mind. By just *breathing*, I learned to heal myself. You don't need to wait for a pharmaceutical company to formulate the next "magic pill." You don't need a celebrity to tell you that a particular fitness program will transform you inside and out. You don't need to be rushed to the emergency room to get a wake up call. On Wall Street, insider secrets provide investors with strategies for profit based on the knowledge of people who have been in the trenches. I've been in the trenches. I almost lost everything in the most profound way. The smartest people learn from others' mistakes. Learn from mine. *You* are your biggest investment. The best "insider secret" I can give you to maximize your investment is this:

Prevention is more important than the cure. With this book, you can focus on your specific needs through my strategically-designed yoga routines. It's also an "initiation" into a simple yogic approach to life that will bring you greater happiness, well-being and peace of mind.

Awareness is the first step to healing. And an open mind is the first step to awareness. Have an open mind as you turn these pages...

AND BREATHE... BREATHE... BREATHE.

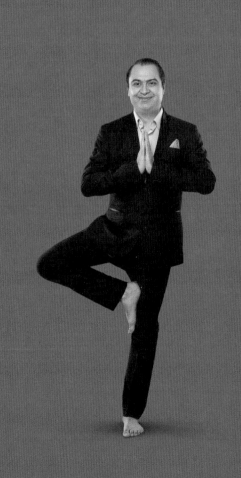

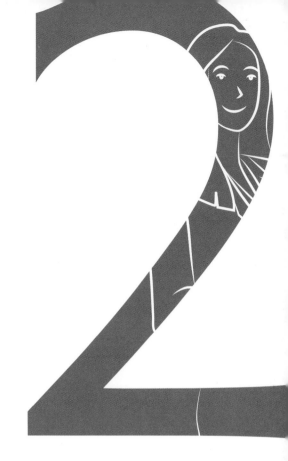

BULLS AND BEARS

Are You a Wall Street Personality?

"For every effort, there needs to be surrender and vice-versa.
With each inhale, rise your body against the gravity.
With each exhale, release it to Mother Earth."

- GuruNanda

ON WALL STREET, THERE ARE TWO MAIN TYPES OF INVESTORS.

A "bull" is someonewho is optimistic and believes that stock prices will go up. A "bear" is pessimistic, believing that stock prices are going to drop. Both types are strategic and both make money. When we think of a Wall Street broker or investor, generally a buttoned-up, well-dressed man or woman with a briefcase and a quick, purposeful stride comes to mind. These people are fast-moving, fast-talking and fast-thinking. They are in perpetual motion, either physically, mentally or most often, both. However, even if you don't work on Wall Street, you very well might be a Wall Street personality. Care to find out?

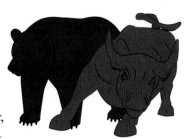

1. I am most satisfied when I'm multi-tasking. If I'm not doing two or more things at once, I feel bored.
Agree. Disgree.

2. I have a difficult time falling asleep, staying asleep or both. I simply have too much on my mind.
Agree. Disgree.

3. I would rather grab a fast food lunch or quick snack, and eat at my desk or on the run than waste time sitting properly at a table.
Agree. Disgree.

4. I can't get through an afternoon without at least one double espresso or energy drink.
Agree. Disgree.

5. I wish I had more of a social life, but I feel guilty if I'm not being productive.
Agree. Disgree.

6. Hobbies? I honestly don't have hobbies anymore.
Agree. Disgree.

7. At least one or more of my personal relationships has suffered because I work too hard or am trying to get too much done all the time.
Agree. Disgree.

8. I haven't taken a vacation in what seems like forever.
Agree. Disgree.

9. I feel a general sense of anxiety.
Agree. Disgree.

10. I don't have time for exercise or I exercise compulsively.
Agree. Disgree.

11. Traffic and bad drivers literally make my blood boil. I have a hard time restraining myself from honking or swearing.
Agree. Disgree.

12. I can't remember the last time I just did nothing.
Agree. Disgree.

13. Right now, I am not breathing deeply.
Agree. Disgree.

If you answered "Agree" to five or more of these statements, then you, my friend, are a fellow Wall Street personality.

Forgive the stereotype: you're Type A (but you probably knew that already). In 1959, cardiologists Meyer Friedman and Ray Rosenman did a study revealing that people with Type A personalities run a higher risk of heart disease and high blood pressure than Type B's. As part of the study, they observed the patients in their waiting room. Some chairs were worn down on the front edges and armrests instead of on the backs. The doctors later observed that those chairs were chosen by coronary patients who tended to sit on the edge of the seat, impatiently waiting for their appointments to begin. These patients were angrier and more high-strung overall.

The Wall Street personality actually runs the gamut:

- The entrepreneur, like me, who is coming up with new concepts, making deals or executing strategies - or all three at once.
- The career woman who is determined to break the surprisingly still present glass ceiling.
- The stay-at-home mom or dad who is organizing the entire family's schedule, keeping the house running and making sure that everyone is fed and happy.
- The college student who is overwhelmed with homework while holding down a job to pay off student loans.
- The freelance creative who is juggling many assignments at once and meeting rapid-fire deadlines.
- The actor or actress who is endlessly competing and honing his or her craft in an increasingly cutthroat industry.

Our world is filled with more Wall Street personalities than ever. Many of us spend far too much time hunched over our laptops, cellphones and tablets. This type of "desk posture" causes shallow breathing that's high in the chest instead of deep into our diaphragm where our breath should reside.

OTHER ENEMIES OF FREE BREATH:

- Neck Ties = strangle your throat
- High Heels = keep you off balance
- Tight Belts = compress your stomach
- Snug Clothing = suffocates the entire body

All of these enemies of breath cause stress. Stress is natural. For animals, stress is *necessary*. A lion aggressively hunts its prey - for example, a deer. The deer protectively runs for its life. Similarly, for our earliest ancestors, this "Fight or Flight Mode" meant running or physically fighting when their lives were in danger.

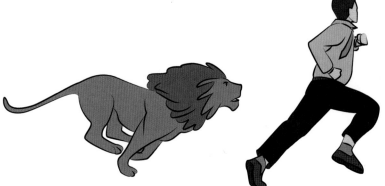

With this type of organic, "healthy" stress, more oxygen, blood and glucose to travel to the extremities. Breathing rate increases, airways open and pupils widen so sight and judgment improve. These are the positive attributes of stress and serve to help successfully meet goals.

Animals forget about a stressful situation once it's over. As humans, though, our recall and memories can sear stress into our psyches, ultimately taking a toll on our physical and emotional health. Prolonged stress can become chronic. For example, a rise in blood pressure while jogging is normal but, if your blood pressure rises constantly because of stress, disease can set in.

Road rage is a perfect example. You're stuck in terrible traffic or someone cuts you off. Your anger spikes and you go into that "Fight or Flight Mode" when your heart beats faster, and extra blood and glucose are pumped to muscles. But your seatbelt is keeping you from releasing your stress the way exercise would. This type of constriction, if persistent, can lead to high blood pressure, hypertension and even diabetes.

Studies reveal that stress can also impair our immune system, leading to everything from colds to cancer.

Wall Street personalities are generally more prone to:

- Heart disease
- Hypertension
- Diabetes

- Depression
- Autoimmune diseases

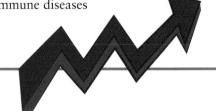

We all know that too much stress is bad. In yogic terms, stress reduces our PRANA. Prana means "life force" in Sanskrit. *Balance* is what is required to keep prana at its peak. The left side of our brain is the logical and calculative side. The right side of our brain is the creative and intuitive side. Wall Street personalities more readily use the left side of the brain, throwing off the healthy balance.

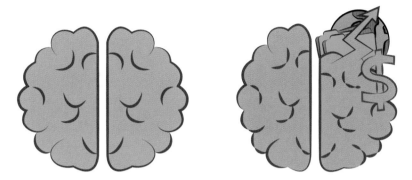

Beloved pets, like our dogs and cats, can teach us much about balance. They stretch their bodies when they wake up. They eat when they are hungry and lap up water when they are thirsty. They take naps when they are tired. They smell and observe their surroundings. And they gaze at us without judgment or criticism. How similar are you to your pet? Have we lost the best parts of our animal instinct?

Prana is about balance and it's the result of this holistic combination:

BREATH - Yoga asanas (poses) and yogic breathing allow for an uninterrupted flow of oxygen and nutrients.

OPTIMISM - Positive thinking builds on itself. The more you see the glass as half full, the more you will have to drink because your attitude will lead you to approach life that way.

NUTRITION - Eating foods in their most natural, organic state *and in moderation* gives your body exactly what it needs.

DEEDS - Right action and generosity create good karmic energy. Simply, what goes around comes around.

B.O.N.D.

In financial terms, a bond is an instrument of indebtedness of the bond issuer to the holders, otherwise known as a loan. In the case of prana, you are both the bond issuer and holder. Every bond has a lifetime, and so do you. Like I mentioned in Chapter 1, *you are investing in yourself*. And if you do that properly, with conscious effort, the returns will be off-the-charts!

The principals of financial investing change as the financial climate changes. The principals of yoga have been in place for thousands of years and will *never* change. There are eight of them. They are easy to remember and follow. And they are the key to your prana - your life force - your B.O.N.D. Don't be put off by language that might sound "lofty." These principals are all very basic and attainable.

THE EIGHT PRINCIPALS OF YOGA are also called "limbs" because they branch out from each other, creating a "tree" that's the foundation of well-being.

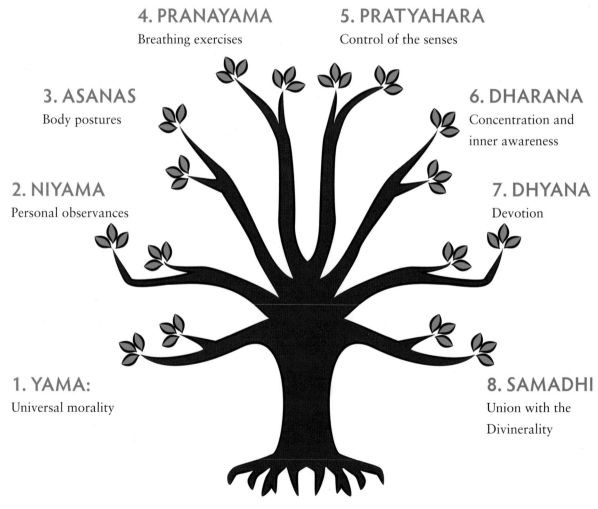

4. PRANAYAMA
Breathing exercises

5. PRATYAHARA
Control of the senses

3. ASANAS
Body postures

6. DHARANA
Concentration and inner awareness

2. NIYAMA
Personal observances

7. DHYANA
Devotion

1. YAMA:
Universal morality

8. SAMADHI
Union with the Divinerality

Don't slam the book shut yet! I'm not telling you who or what your "Divine" - or God - is. You might not even believe in a higher power. **In yogic terms, the Divine is who you are inside.** Yoga literally means "union," so by practicing, you will become more connected to yourself. Being more connected to yourself will give you a sense of peace and calm that you never knew. I speak from what I know.

Wall Street Yoga will focus on the first three yogic principals:

YAMA "universal morality," is our attitude toward the world around us. Yamas are broken down into five "wise characteristics." They are not "Do's" and "Don't's" but instead guidelines to *being* that ultimately contribute to the health and happiness of everyone around us:

1. Ahimsa - Compassion for all living things
2. Satya - Commitment to truthfulness
3. Asteya - Not stealing when it comes to material items *and* other people's time, efforts and trust
4. Brahmacharya - Sense control by harnessing our sexual energy or animal instinct, and using it in a productive way
5. Aparigraha - Neutralizing the desire to acquire and hoard wealth

NIYAMA represents our attitude toward ourselves. Niyamas are "rules" prescribed for personal observation. Niyamas create a "soulfulness" that translates to the way we walk around in the world:

1. Saucha - Keep your body and thoughts clean. In Chapter 7, you'll be inspired to pare down the excess while you pare down your body with better nutrition.
2. Samtosha - Be grateful for what you have rather than crying and yearning for more.
3. Tapas - Follow your goals and pursuits enthusiastically instead of compulsively.
4. Svadhyaya - Self-study, which teaches us to be centered and non-reactive.
5. Ishvara Pranidhana - Celebrate the spiritual by understanding that there is a force greater than ourselves. Let go of expectations and the notion that you can control everything. **Expectations reduce joy.**

ASANAS make up the third yogic principal. **Asanas are the yoga poses.** This book will give you different series of poses based on what you need in your life, whether:

* You have problems sleeping.
* Your back hurts.
* Your blood sugar levels or blood pressure is high.
* You feel depressed.
* You get crazy when you drive.

Though each series varies, every series provides three physical, emotional and spiritual benefits:
1. Strength to tackle the obstacles of life with vigor and power.
2. Flexibility to be malleable in situations by dropping your ego to attain your goals.
3. Balance so you can live without getting into extreme situations that are unproductive and unhealthy.

The eight limbs of yoga are really about karma. If you're doing right - if your *attitude* is right - right karma comes back in the form of positive energy. Asanas will give you strength, flexibility and balance, physically, emotionally and spiritually. Regular meditation gives you the power to stop stress *at will* so that you will be more open to right thoughts, attitudes and actions.

Does all this sound like a tall order that requires time and energy you don't have? Guess what?

WALL STREET YOGA TAKES AS LITTLE AS 14 MINUTES A DAY!

2 minutes of meditation in the morning

+

2 minutes of meditation in the evening

+

10 minutes of simple asanas (poses)

=

14 MINUTES TO TRANSFORM YOUR LIFE

This book will give you 10-MINUTE YOGA ROUTINES with SIMPLE POSES for:

- Morning
- Bedtime
- Anxiety and depression
- Weight loss
- Heart health
- Back pain and sciatica
- Car/Driving stress

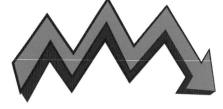

In addition to the main poses in each routine, you'll get bonus poses (because everyone likes a bonus). They might be a little more challenging, but as with every pose, I will walk you through them step-by-step. Video demonstrations of all the poses can be found on my website at www.gurunanda.com.

Make sure you do your bonus poses before CORPSE POSE, traditionally known as Shavasana, which is the final pose in every routine (except in Chapter 10's Yoga for Driving). This pose is the golden end to your yoga practice. After moving through asanas, Corpse Pose is a form of surrender and self-acceptance, and it provides a few precious moments of "resting in peace" in the most positive sense. It's a reward - skipping it is like forgoing salary after a full day's work!

CORPSE "SHAVASANA" POSE

CORPSE "SHAVASANA" POSE

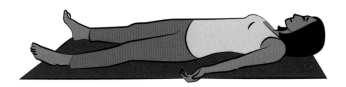

a. Lie on your back. Your feet should be hip distance apart and your arms are by your sides. Your palms are facing up.

b. Close your eyes.

c. Take 3 deep breaths through your *nose only*. If you are congested, breathe through your mouth so that it's comfortable for you.

d. Start relaxing. Progressively, from your toes up to your shins… knees… thighs… hips… stomach… chest… arms… neck… and forehead. You will finally feel like your entire body is heavy and melted into the floor. Your breath will become shallow - that's okay.

e. Pretend that you are looking at your body from above.
Be in that awareness state for ONE MINUTE - you are a spectator, not in your body itself. If you decide to stay in the pose for longer, even better!
In my opinion, one minute of Corpse Pose is equal to 10 minutes of restful sleep.

f. Gently roll onto your right side and slowly sit up.

You don't need to do all the routines every day. At the very least, pick one routine a day. You might find one that works best for you overall. You may feel that bookending your day with yoga in the morning and evening gives you the most rewards (this is my personal favorite way to incorporate yoga). Or you might like to mix it up, depending on what's going on in your life. That being said, the meditation is non-negotiable. You'll learn why in Chapter 4, but suffice to say, meditation changed my life and I guarantee that the 2 minutes, twice a day will change yours.

The trick to reaping yoga's profound benefits is regularity, but it's a trick that you'll learn like kids' magic. With every 14 minutes of Wall Street Yoga, you will look forward to the next 14 minutes. Those 14 minutes will quickly become a necessary part of your life because you will feel good! Wall Street Yoga becomes completely natural.

A very successful colleague of mine told me he met a girl at the airport. He was prattling on and on to her about his business and lifestyle, trying to impress her. She was flying to see friends from college. It wasn't really a trip she could afford, but she was so excited to just go to the beach with her pals. He mentioned his fancy car. She mentioned her beautiful garden. She was learning how to play the guitar. He couldn't remember the last time he learned something new. When they parted, my colleague realized that he had been working for decades just to do *one* of the activities the woman regularly enjoyed. He realized he didn't have to *work* to do them. They had been available to him all along.

As a Wall Street personality, your stress can radiate out in your life. It is a cycle I caused that led to not only my unhappiness, but the unhappiness of everyone around me.

MAELSTROM OF MISERY

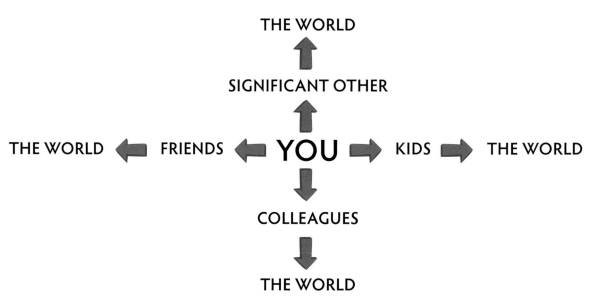

You are not a bull or a bear. You are a human being. Ask yourself, did you come to earth to enjoy living here or are you in a "mad rush" to finish? Do you keep putting off your dreams until…

- You get that promotion?
- You get married?
- Your kids graduate?
- You retire?

As far as we know, we are on this earth for a finite amount of time. Take a breather - literally - and decide how you want to live.

Then, take 14 minutes and make a change.

ENJOY LIFE NOW.

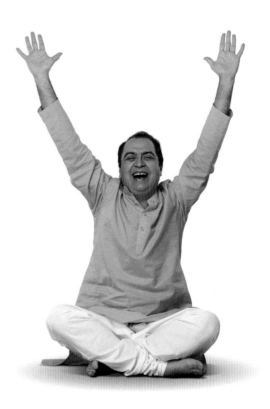

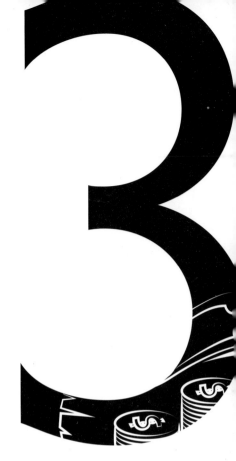

CAPITAL
GAINS

The Science Behind Yoga's Rewards

"Yoga protects your most valuable investment: your body."

- GuruNanda

CAPITAL GAINS ARE INVESTMENT REWARDS.

They're the profits you enjoy when the selling price of an asset exceeds the purchase price. Yoga is all about capital gains. You get *so much* out of putting in so little. And where monetary investments can lead to capital loss, **yoga reaps only profits**. It's a sure-fire win.

People win and lose in the stock market, because no one can really figure out the science behind investing. But yoga's significant and perpetual wins *are* science-based. In fact, yoga is a 5,000-year-old science!

Here is the simple scientific explanation for yoga: Yoga releases beta endorphins in the brain which elevate mood and relieve pain. It acts like the drug morphine, but you don't need a prescription. You *should* (and I believe, *will*) get addicted to yoga.

Yoga is based on this basic formula: P.U.R.E.

PERSPIRATION

URINATION

RESPIRATION

EXCRETION

The body works on **the P.U.R.E. System** to eradicate everyday toxins being poured and infused into our bodies from stress, aggression, overwork, pollution and medication. Without yoga, the **P.U.R.E.** System doesn't work. For example:

All FOUR ways of natural toxin release are obstructed = P.U.R.E. The solution: A YOGIC WAY OF LIFE.

- Exercise = Perspiration
- Sufficient water intake = Urination
- Pranayama during yoga and meditation = Respiration
- Conscientious eating + hydration + yoga = Excretion

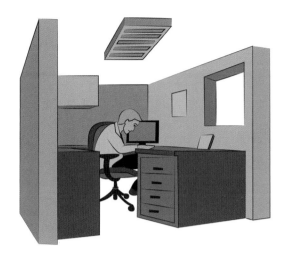

- The office-goer slogs from a stuffy car in oppressive traffic to an air-conditioned office. No real movement or fresh air = ~~PERSPIRATION.~~

- He drinks coffee in the morning, soda at lunch, an energy drink in the afternoon and a cocktail with dinner. No water = ~~URINATION~~

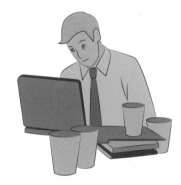

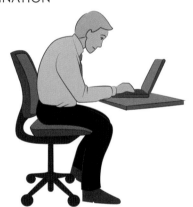

- Hunched over his desk, his laptop, his cellphone and/or his tablet, his diaphragm is constricted. Add the stress he feels at work causes shallow, anxious breathing. A lack of deep breaths = ~~RESPIRATION~~

- A drive-through breakfast sandwich, a fast food lunch and a dinner eaten hastily by the TV is combined with a lack of water intake. Bad nutrition + dehydration = ~~EXCRETION~~

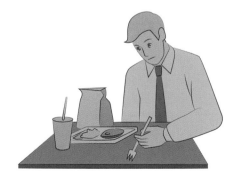

For most Wall Street personalities, our lungs only perform at 15-20% of their capacity. You can actually double that number by doing yogic breathing.

When I first started doing yoga, a teacher told me, "You're doing great exercise, but you're not doing yoga, because yoga is not about just moving your hands and feet. Real yoga is about breathing." Many people believe that if you're doing poses, you're doing yoga, but you're not *breathing*. You're just *moving*. The goal of yoga is not to shape your body into a pretzel. The difference between a stretch and an asana (pose) is that in an asana, we move with the breath as one unified body and mind.

BREATHING IS LIFE. One of the eight limbs of yoga is **PRANAYAMA**, also known as **breathing exercises.** In Sanskrit, "Prana" means life force or vital energy, particularly, the breath. "Ayama" means to extend or draw out.

> # PRAYANAMA =
> ## "extension of the prana or breath"
> ## or
> ## "extension of the life force"

Pranayama yoga goes hand-in-hand with the asanas.

I learned that to get the true benefits of yoga, you must breathe calmness into every move. When you do yoga properly, not forcefully, you will breathe and stretch in poses that bring the extra oxygen and nutrients to your body, helping clear out the toxins at the cellular level. More nutrients permeate the cell membranes, into the cytoplasm. So, we end up with cleaner, more disease-free cells that actually have the potential to cure themselves and regenerate. Breathing in the poses allows you to absorb the full benefits of each movement. It's the payoff and, as Wall Street personalities, we all like it when work pays off.

YOGA BREATH BASICS

Here is how to get the maximum benefits from your yogic breathing:

- Breathe through your nose only.
- Inhale *slowly*.
- Your exhale should be a little longer than your inhale, if possible.

Note: If you have a cold or are congested, it's okay to breathe through your mouth, so that you're comfortable. As with all yoga, do what you can. **Just remember to BREATHE.**

As an inventor and a perpetual science "student," I am a firm supporter of modern medicine. Modern medicine - from antibiotics to surgery to imaging, plus assured balanced nutrition due to irrigation and agricultural advancement - has helped increase our average life span from 40 to 80 years. However, new complex-lifestyle diseases like diabetes, hypertension, heart disease, stroke and cancer, have been growing. And stress plays a big part in this pandemic. Consequently, the medical industry is progressively accepting the importance of integrating mind-body practices with Western methodologies, and doctors are increasingly recommending yoga.

Yoga is simply great preventative "medicine" because our bodies are intrinsically self-healing machines.

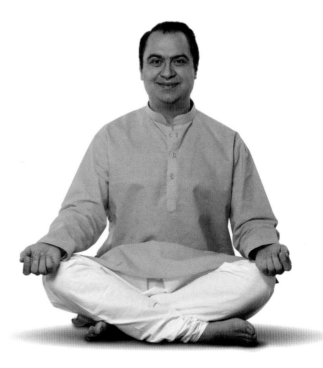

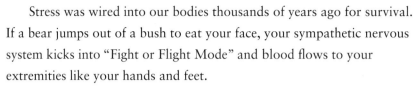

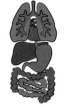

Stress was wired into our bodies thousands of years ago for survival. If a bear jumps out of a bush to eat your face, your sympathetic nervous system kicks into "Fight or Flight Mode" and blood flows to your extremities like your hands and feet.

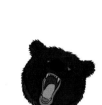

Your heart rate and blood pressure rise and non-emergency organs like the stomach, intestines, kidneys and reproductive organs get deprived of critical blood flow. This was all designed for physical exertion.

But nowadays, fights with bears are few and far between, so we are experiencing stress without the necessary physical outlet. In our modern culture, this unhealthy state gets activated in our bodies about ten times a day. Man-eating bears have been replaced by man-eating bosses, tigers by traffic jams, and crocodiles by crabby customer service.

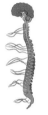

Yogic breathing activates our parasympathetic nervous system, which is just a science-y word for the part of our nervous system that slows us down.

Yoga is to stress like water is to fire.

When you do yoga with proper breathing, stress eases the heart rate and blood circulation goes back to the non-emergency organs for better body function and overall health.

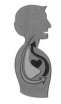

Yoga affects our cells, too. Certain cells in our body get deprived of oxygen and vital nutrients due to our desktop lifestyles. Instead of chasing prey, we sit at our computers, using only a fraction of our lung capacity. Yogic breathing can dramatically increase this, pushing oxygen through the body to better permeate our deprived cells.

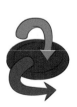

As oxygen is pushed into the cell walls, carbon dioxide waste and toxins are pushed out of the cell with equal force, helping the cells cure themselves and remain disease-free.

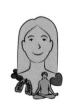

YOGA = HAPPY, HEALTHY CELLS = HAPPY, HEALTHY BODY.

THE END

The diaphragm is the only muscle in the body that's both voluntary and involuntary (unlike the heart, which is involuntary, versus the hand, which is voluntary). Your breath is a connector between your conscious and subconscious mind. By regulating your breath, which consciously moves the diaphragm, you can train yourself to control some key physiological functions.

Here's one of my favorite analogies about doing yoga: If you want the best tasting toast and your toaster has six heat settings, set the heat to 3. At 2, your toast will come out too soft. At 4, your toast will end up burnt. Yoga needs to be practiced for a certain period of time to reap the best gains. I want to help you make perfectly delicious toast, so to speak.

THE WALL STREET YOGA "RX"
2 MINUTES OF MEDITATION, TWICE A DAY,
PLUS 10 MINUTES OF POSES.
14 MINUTES A DAY. THAT'S IT!

If you really want to experience transformation, here are more yoga-inspired preventative "prescriptions":

- **LISTEN TO MUSIC** - The vibrations created by music help heal the body's chakras (energy points), connecting the conscious with the subconscious. If your find driving stressful, then listen to calm and joyful music instead of loud rock that aggravates your already-agitated sympathetic nervous system.

- **DANCE** - Dancing lets you free your focus from the outside world. Find a private space, turn on your favorite music, and dance with your eyes closed. Dance as if today is the ultimate day. Don't worry about feeling foolish! After one full song, lay in Corpse Pose to absorb the total body goodness.

- **CREATE** - Activate the artist inside you. When you paint or draw, the colors reflect and express your mood. Cooking new and creative dishes allows for fresh tastes. Gardening lets you enjoy seeing the fruits of your labors.

- **LAUGH** - It's been said that, "Laughter is the best medicine." I say, "Those who do **laughter yoga** need *no* medicine." Did you know that our body doesn't recognize the difference between fake and real laughing? In Chapter 5, I will introduce you to laughter yoga and gibberish that can melt away your stress and help you tackle challenging situations.

- **CUDDLE** - Oxytocin is a hormone that has been shown to reduce stress-related physical damage. It relaxes the brain and regenerates the heart from stress damage. Oxytocin is commonly called "The

Cuddle Hormone." Positive voluntary social interactions with the people you love releases oxytocin, creating a buffer and resistance to stress.

• **INTERACT** - Simple, daily social interactions are natural mood boosters. A water cooler conversation about last night's favorite TV show, a visit to the dog park where other pet lovers gather, or a pleasant chat at the grocery store check-out line all lighten our stress load. I'm not big on coffee, but my favorite latte spot is what I call "the oxytocin station," where easy, social interactions produce benefits that outweigh the caffeine negatives. That's a net gain.

I am physical proof that the science behind yoga is infinitely rewarding:

- I lost 40 pounds.
- I stopped snoring.
- My cholesterol and blood pressure are both lower.
- My chronic lower back pain has subsided.
- My headaches are dramatically reduced.
- I don't suffer from any more panic attacks.
- I am off almost all meds.

A tortoise takes 4 breaths per minute.
Average life span: 150 years.

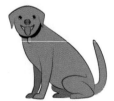

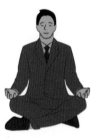

A human takes 15 breaths per minute.
Average life span: 80 years.

A dog takes over 40 breaths per minute.
Average life span: 15 years.

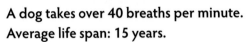

BREATHE LIKE A TORTOISE AND LIVE LONGER.

We have become conditioned not to value free stuff. But yoga is a free gift from our ancestors that has extraordinary value. The capital gains are immeasurable.

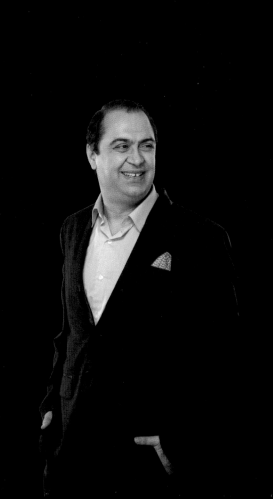

LONG-TERM TERM INVESTING

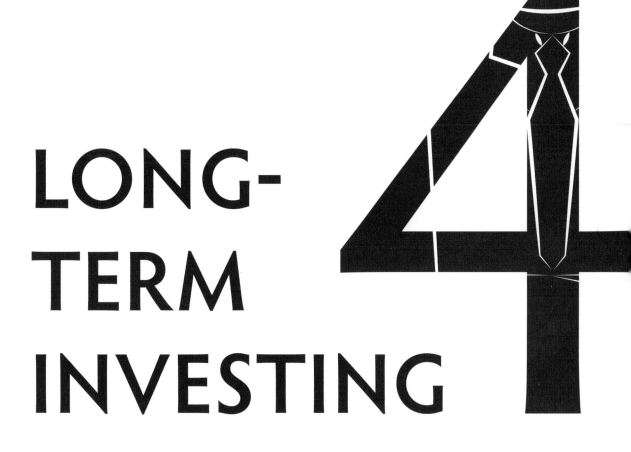

Coming Out Ahead with Meditation

"Breathing is the single most important part of yoga."

- GuruNanda

TRENDS DRIVE THE STOCK MARKET, BUT LONG-TERM INVESTING

has traditionally been known as safer than chasing hot tips for quick profit. Think about the fable of the tortoise that moved slow and steady to beat the hare to victory. Wall Street personalities need to learn how to move more slowly so as not to physically and emotionally burn out. Meditation is the first step to the long race that is life. It will get you in touch with **PRAKRUTI**, the universe's primal motive force, perpetually available to all of us for a more deeply satisfying existence. With meditation, even though you are *still*, you are moving forward, but it's in a meaningful and deliberate way as opposed to the rush-rush-rush to get there, wherever "there" is.

Research has established that a few aware deep breaths and a couple minutes of meditation, done properly, can reduce blood pressure and provide positive relaxation. Meditation has been scientifically proven to help alleviate and/or manage stress-induced conditions like aches and pains, depression, anxiety, insomnia, drug abuse, high blood pressure, asthma, allergies... even cancer.

THE MAGIC MEDITATION 30

1. It lowers heart rate and high blood pressure.
2. It increases blood flow and promotes circulation.
3. It improves exercise tolerance and athletic performance.
4. By increasing the serotonin level, it's an anxiety-reducer and mood-booster.
5. It decreases muscle tension.
6. It helps alleviate premenstrual syndrome (PMS) symptoms.
7. It supports post-operative healing.
8. It helps to strengthen the immune system and combat virus activity.
9. It helps with weight loss.
10. It makes skin more radiant and luminous.
11. It can lower cholesterol levels.
12. It helps soothe headaches and migraines.
13. It enhances brain function, focus, concentration and creativity.
14. It helps balance the endocrine system.
15. It aids fertility by reducing stress.
16. It improves relationships, social interactions and intimacy.
17. It boosts sexual performance, endurance and flexibility.
18. It helps quell fears and control phobias.
19. By building willpower, it helps eradicate bad habits and addictions, including smoking.
20. It helps you develop stronger intuition.
21. It fosters patience.
22. It helps you ignore petty issues and see the larger picture.
23. It improves perceptual ability and motor skills.
24. It has been known to increase job satisfaction.
25. It helps alleviate insomnia.
26. It reduces road rage.
27. It makes you a better and more compassionate listener.
28. It gives you a deeper understanding of yourself.
29. It helps you live in the present moment.
30. It promotes peace of mind and happiness.

As Wall Street personalities, we have trouble quieting our minds, so mantra-based meditation is, in my opinion, the best type of meditation for us, especially when coupled with meditative breathing. It lets you keep the traffic of thoughts flowing - good and bad - without any self-judgment while helping you focus on a positive affirmation.

Why have mantra? It's a vehicle. Our brain gets thousands and thousands of thoughts every minute. By giving it *one* job to do - *repeating the mantra* - the mind will have a specific focus. Your mind will become so trained to focus on your positive mantra that it will literally press the "delete button" on negative thoughts, erasing them from your conscious and subconscious mind.

There is a huge difference between **concentration** and **meditation**. Concentration is tiresome focus of mind. Meditation is freedom. It's allowing all ideas and thoughts to flow with absolutely zero resistance. Use your mantra as a boat to glide across the ocean of ever-invading thoughts.

The traditional general mantra I suggest when you are starting mantra-based meditation is "**OM NIROGAYA NAMAH.**"

The universal sound "**OM**" has three parts:
1. **Ohhh** = the Creator = the organs below our navel (kidneys, urinary tract, reproductive organs)
2. **Ahhh** = the Preserver = the organs between the neck and navel (heart, liver)
3. **Ammm** = The Super Creator = the organs above our neck (thyroid, sinus, brain, pituitary)

"**OM**" has often been referred to as "the white light." White light contains all seven colors of the rainbow. When you chant "Om," your body is infused with all seven colors, integrating all life's energy.

"Nirogaya Namah" means "health without any disease" or "The Divine will dilute all diseases." In yoga, when we say "Om Nirogaya Namah," we are talking about physical, emotional *and* spiritual health.

Or you can adopt a more personal mantra. This will be the sound of the universe that is specific to *you*. A personal mantra can really enhance your meditative process. As you continue meditating, it will work more and more and more to calm you, center you, and bring you peace and joy. Since your mantra will settle deep into your subconscious, eventually you will *instantly relax* when you say it. Just the thought of it will calm you down. It's the opposite of how the thought of an irate boss or an angry significant other can rile you up. The mantra sounds better, right?

My first personal mantra was "I am strong, healthy and decisive," because in my subconscious, I was not any of those things. To figure out *your* personal mantra, write down the areas where you feel you are lacking. Then, turn those around to positive, optimistic aspirations.

Do you want to be...

- Focused
- Creative
- Relaxed
- Adventurous

- Powerful
- Open-minded
- Optimistic
- Kind

- Present
- Connected
- Honest
- Grateful

Don't share your personal mantra. Keep it pure. And when you find the mantra that works for you, don't change it. The more you meditate, and the more you focus on it, the more powerful it will become for you.

Since Wall Street personalities are always strategizing and planning, you will notice that your innovation will kick into gear when you begin meditating. Hundreds of product ideas would pop into my head. When I first started meditating, I would be tempted to open my eyes and put my thoughts on paper, afraid I would forget a golden nugget. But here's even more meditation "magic": if the thought is strong enough, then it automatically comes back when you're finished meditating, If it's not strong enough, it fades away. Meditation has an "auto-filter," separating the wheat from the chaff.

Most importantly, with meditation, patience and perseverance are key. Many people quit early because they want a quick "result." Remember the yamas and niyamas - leave your desire out of the equation!

2 MINUTES, TWICE A DAY IS ALL THE MEDITATION YOU NEED!
IN THAT 2 MINUTES, YOU CAN REPEAT YOUR MANTRA **108** TIMES.
Why 108?

- In India, astrophysics, astrology and spiritualism have always been connected. Around 5000 B.C., Indians calculated that the diameter of the sun multiplied **108** times is the distance from the earth to the sun. Coincidentally, the diameter of the moon multiplied **108** times gives you the distance from the earth to the moon. The cosmic ratio of the closest two planets are thought to influence earth and human fortunes.

- There are 54 letters in the Sanskrit alphabet. Each has masculine and feminine, Shiva and Shakti. 54 x 2 = 108.

- The chakras, our energy centers, have a total of **108** energy lines converging to form the heart chakra.

My reason for repeating my mantra **108** times? **IT WORKS**.

Normally, meditation is done with the actions of the sun - when it comes up and when it goes down. You don't have to be that specific with your meditation time, but try to **START AND END YOUR DAY WITH MEDITATION.** Do your evening meditation 3-4 hours *before* bedtime so you don't stimulate your mind right before sleep. Use it to let go of your day and ease into your night.

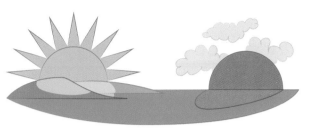

10 SIMPLE STEPS FOR MANTRA-BASED MEDITATION

1. Find a quiet space. When I started doing meditation, I sat in the back seat of my car in the parking lot at my office. Try to meditate at the same time and place.

2. Sit comfortably, but keep your spine straight so you don't fall asleep. If you're on the floor using a mat or blanket, sit in a cross-legged position with your hands resting on your knees, palms up.

3. Close your eyes.

4. Chant "Om" 3 times with deep breaths in between, slowly releasing the sounds "Ohh," "Ahh" and "Amm," which brings your awareness from the organs below the navel to the mid-section to the head.

5. Say the universal mantra "Om Nirogaya Namah" or your personal mantra twice out loud. Quiet to a whisper, repeating it over and over. Then, start thinking it rather than saying it. The silent recitation will help silence your mind.

6. When other thoughts come in, let them flow. Just *very gently* bring your awareness back to your mantra. You may become aware of noises you don't usually hear, like birds outside or a bike whizzing past or the laundry whirring in your house. Let it in, then let it go. Those noises will fade.

7. Set a soft alarm for 2 minutes or have someone gently touch you on the shoulder.

8. Take a deep breath.

9. Rub your hands together. Place your naturally heated hands on your eyes, then your face.

10. Put your palms together in Prayer Position at the center of your chest. This area represents your heart. Bow your body slightly forward and feel a moment of gratitude, then open your eyes.

Prayer Position is traditionally known as "Namaste." You do not need to have a religious affiliation for Namaste. The gesture merely acknowledges The Divine spark in each of us that is located in the heart chakra. During our yoga practice, whether in the poses, after the poses or after meditation, Prayer Position/Namaste helps us connect deeper with that chakra. When we live from the heart chakra, we can better connect with others and with life itself. A slight bow with Namaste depicts a surrender of the ego in an act of appreciation for who you are and all those around you.

Remember, when you meditate, your thoughts and feelings will come and go - love, sadness, even anger. Don't shun or stop those thoughts or feelings. Meditation can initially stir things up before you release and find a state of bliss. Skeptical? Try it. Let your mind wander during meditation. As soon as you remember your mantra, very gently go back to it. Don't force it. Be a kind and gentle "boss" to yourself. You will naturally get back to your "job" meditating.

When your meditation is complete, move on. I guarantee that in the short-term, you will feel more relaxed, but not sleepy. If you fall asleep during meditation, that means you are not well rested (Chapter 11 will help you with insomnia and sleep disorders). Good meditation will energize you in a content way. It's like restarting your computer when it's sluggish or acting up. Long-term - that's where the rewards really pay off, because meditation teaches you that everything is a moment. What's "good" now, won't be "good" forever. What's "bad" now, won't be "bad" forever. You can't always change circumstances, but you can always change your *attitude* toward those circumstances.

Life is a wave-like pattern of change. Yoga and meditation teach you to ride those waves with flexibility and an open mind. Most importantly, stick with it. The process is like peeling an onion. Every time you meditate, you will peel away another layer, uncovering more and more about yourself that will move you to a more peaceful, satisfied, happy state. Give meditation the same type of shot you would anything important in your life and I promise,

THE INVALUABLE RESULTS WILL COME.

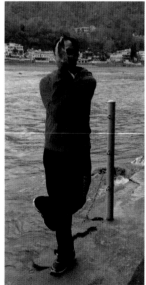

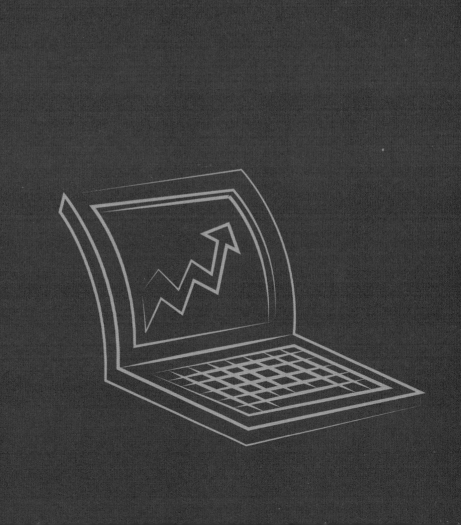

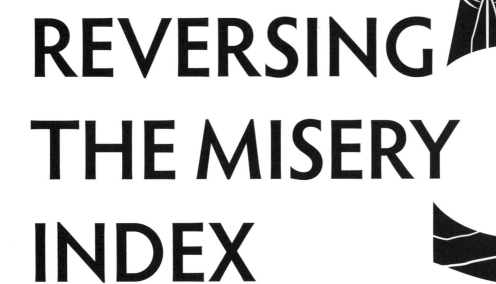

REVERSING THE MISERY INDEX

Yoga for Depression and Anxiety

"In life, 'Fake it til you make it' works with laughter yoga. The sound and feeling of your own happiness will inspire *true* happiness."

- GuruNanda

ON WALL STREET, THE MISERY INDEX IS A MEASURE OF ECONOMIC WELL-BEING FOR A SPECIFIED ECONOMY, using unemployment and inflation rates.

An increasing Misery Index means a worsening economic climate. A decreasing Misery Index means things are getting better. In yogic terms, we work toward a steadily improving "personal index."

Although we have come far in so many ways - from technology to consumer products, transportation to communication - the fundamental nature of mankind has remained the same. We have a great many positive attributes as human beings, but we can't deny negative feelings like jealousy, hatred, competition, impatience and anxiety. Traffic, a bad job, discontented relationships, dysfunctional family, financial problems and perpetual global crises seep into our psyches in a way that makes us want to hold our breath or scream out loud. These feelings are exacerbated by instantaneous expression: Facebook bullying, a "break-up" via text message, or an e-mail from a nasty boss who expects an answer right away.

In business, whenever an employee made a mistake, I got very upset and wanted to yell and shout. Now, I laugh at those emotions that would otherwise manifest themselves as pain in my neck and shoulders. Ancient yoga can't guarantee a stress-free life, but it can show us the way to controlling our own anxiety and depression levels.

During high stress situations, a hormone called **cortisol** is released that can ultimately cause:

- Bone loss
- Low immunity
- Collagen loss
- Impotency
- Obesity
- High blood pressure

Laughter, when done in a yogic format, *regulates* cortisol. Laughter yoga also releases **endorphins**, which have an analgesic and "feel good" effect. Endorphins help with:

- Mediating depression
- Reducing panic attacks
- Lowering blood pressure
- Boosting immunity
- Anti-aging

Laughter isn't a cure-all, but research continues to show that it has exceptionally valuable benefits, including:

MOOD IMPROVEMENT - According to the Centers for Disease Control and Prevention (CDC), an estimated 1 in 10 adults suffers from some form of depression. Laughter yoga helps calm anxiety and, most simply, makes you feel better - right away. I took anti-depressants until I started laughing like a yogi.

TENSION AND PAIN RELIEF - Laughter energizes circulation and relaxes the muscles, helping alleviate physical symptoms caused by stress, like headaches, back pain and muscle stiffness. Laughter prompts the body to produce oxytocin, which acts as a natural painkiller.

ORGAN STIMULATION - Laughter increases oxygen intake, and gets the lungs, heart and muscles going.

IMMUNE SYSTEM ENHANCEMENT - Neuropeptides fight the stress that can cause illness. Laughter releases neuropeptides.

Laughter is also **social booster**. Challenging situations and various types of personalities are easier to deal with when you have a sense of humor - "laugh it off."

THE ANATOMY OF LAUGHTER YOGA

LAUGHTER YOGA at first might seem goofy to you because it is forced laughter, not laughter that comes from watching a funny movie or seeing a silly meme online. It certainly seemed goofy to me. But there is physical science behind laughter yoga. Let's break it down before you try it:

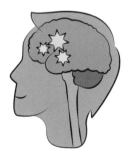

"VERY GOOD! VERY GOOD!" CHANT

As human beings, we all love to be appreciated and rewarded. Dopamine is a chemical that is produced in the brain when we get rewarded. When you appreciate yourself by repeatedly saying phrases like "Very good! Very good! Very good!" you release dopamine, this reward hormone.

CLAPPING

Like feet, the hands have pressure points that connect with other parts of the body. By clapping, you're actually stimulating the acupressure points for focus and better memory.

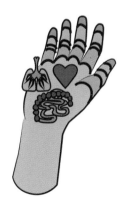

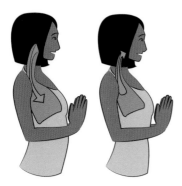

"HO-HO-HA-HA-HA" CHANT + CLAPPING

This combination elevates the "laughter energy." The "H" sound prompts you to use your diaphragm so you breathe and move oxygen, ridding your body of toxins. You're correcting improper breathing with the slightly forceful release of stale gasses stuck in the bottom area of your lungs - the result of being hunched over a desk or laptop, or sitting in traffic. **Always try to laugh more from your stomach and heart, instead of the throat.**

Laughter yoga encompasses the FOUR A'S that foster emotional fulfillment:

1. **A**ppreciation - Be proud of who you are and all that you do.

2. **A**cceptance - Everything you do should be okay, even your mistakes. Don't judge yourself so harshly.

3. **A**ffection - Treat yourself with love, kindness and a sense of playfulness.

4. **A**ttention - Be aware of what you need and make sure that those needs are fulfilled.

When you satisfy the FOUR A's for yourself, you will more easily be able to experience them and share them with those around you. Goodwill and positive relationships are created that way.

Here is a true story: One of my best friends was fired from his longtime job the day he found out that his mother was dying from cancer. At his office, he felt like he was falling apart. He took a moment for himself and went in the restroom. There, he simply went "Ho-ho-ha-ha-ha!" a few times. Mind you, he did not previously practice any yoga. He had only heard about laughter yoga from me, and thought it was pretty silly. But *just the act of making laughter sounds* made him see that this moment would pass. It was just one in a life of many. If he could face his challenges with a smile - even part of the time - he would help himself and everyone around him.

So give it a try. The two routines I recommend are quick and easy. They can be done anywhere when you are feeling anxious, angry or depressed. You can practice them everyday to keep your mood lifted or put them into play during a particularly challenging moment, like an "In case of emergency, break glass" device.

"LAUGHTER YOGA" ROUTINE

*These exercises are best done out loud to reap the full benefits. However, you can always do them silently if you don't want to disturb others (or **you** need privacy).*

SIT ON THE FLOOR. in a cross-legged position or in a basic seated position in a chair. Regardless of where you're sitting, remember to keep your **SPINE STRAIGHT**.

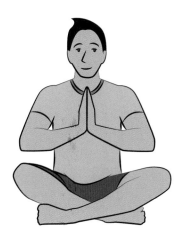

1. THE NAMASTE

a. Bring your palms together in Prayer Position at the center of your chest.

b. Quickly repeat "Ha-ha-ha-ha-ha-ha-ha!" while moving your upper body across your lower body, right to left then left to right. Repeat 2 more times in both directions.

c. Throw your arms in the air in celebration as you say "Ha-ha-ha-ha-ha!" Repeat 2 more times.

d. Put your thumbs and forefingers together by your sides and say "Very good. Very good!" as you move right, then left.

e. Say "Very good!" 1 time toward the middle.

f. Clap your hands to the chant "Ho-ho-ha-ha-ha!" The "ho-ho" is to your left, the "ha-ha-ha" to your right. Repeat 2 more times.

g. Rest your hands on your knees.

h. Breathe and calm down.

2. THE LION

In the jungle of this world, you need to bring the lion inside of you out.

a. Still seated, make "claws" with your hands.

b. Roar like a lion as you move across your body like you are scaring predators. Repeat across your body 2 more times.

c. Throw your arms in the air in celebration as you say "Ha-ha-ha-ha-ha!" Repeat 2 more times.

d. Put your thumbs and forefingers together by your sides and say "Very good! Very good!" as you move right, then left.

e. Say "Very good!" 1 time toward the middle.

f. Clap your hands as you chant "Ho-ho-ha-ha-ha!" The "ho-ho" is to your left, the "ha-ha-ha" to your right. Repeat 2 more times.

g. Rest your hands on your knees.

h. Breathe and calm down.

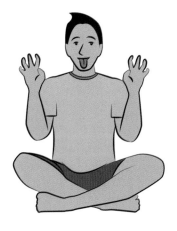

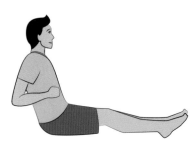

3. THE ROWING

If your world feels like it's coming to an end, you need to row the boat with laughter and a smile.

a. Remain seated. Pretend you are holding one oar with both hands.

b. Row 1 time to the right while saying "Ha!" then once to the left while saying "Ha!" Repeat 4 more times both sides, rowing faster and faster.

c. Throw your arms in the air in celebration as you say "Ha-ha-ha-ha-ha!" Repeat 2 more times.

d. Put your thumbs and forefingers together by your sides and say "Very good! Very good!" as you move right, then left.

e. Say "Very good!" 1 time toward the middle.

f. Clap your hands as you chant "Ho-ho-ha-ha-ha!" The "ho-ho" is to your left, the "ha-ha-ha" to your right. Repeat 2 more times.

g. Rest your hands on your knees.

h. Breathe and calm down.

CORPSE POSE

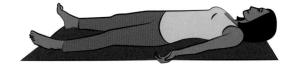

BONUS POSE:

THE JACKPOT

Imagine you've just won the lottery!

a. Stand. Throw your arms up and let your body burst with victory!

b. Laugh "Haaaa! Haaaa!" as you pump your arms, kick your legs, shake your bottom - whatever feels good.

c. Continue for 30 seconds.

d. Stand tall in with your arms loosely by your sides. Your feet should be parallel, hip distance apart. This is Mountain Pose.

e. Breathe and calm down.

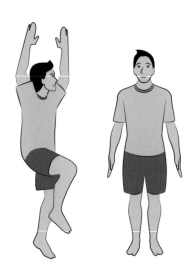

Everyday, you hear things you don't want to hear that create anger and frustration inside of you. If not vented out, this will manifest itself into physical inflexibility, pain and disease. There are two exercises that don't involve laughing, but they are equally helpful in managing anger and anxiety. Again, you can do these anywhere - in your office, in the lunchroom, the restroom, and even in your parked car.

With regular practice, you can train yourself to laugh out negative emotions. You'll actually change the hormone release from one that can cause a stiff neck or painful headache to one that will relax your muscles and your mind.

Remember, laughter yoga does not encourage laughter at other people. That negativity is against the principals of yoga. Once you embrace the yogic way of life, which doesn't include ego or ignorance, your stress levels will automatically go down. Ego and ignorance are the causes of misery.

"MISERY INDEX-REVERSING" ROUTINE

The following exercises are for immediate stress reduction and mood boost. Give yourself a few moments to go "consciously crazy" and clean out the emotional rubbish that no longer serves you. By smashing internal blocks in a safe and FUN way, you'll pump up self-confidence, creativity and focus.

They can be done in a cross-legged position on the floor or in a basic seated position in a chair.
IF YOU'RE IN YOUR CAR, MAKE SURE IT'S PARKED.

1. WILD GIBBERISH

Gibberish releases all negative thoughts, anger and frustration. It breaks up the continuous record repeating itself in our head.

a. Starting in your seated position, let yourself go wild with sounds, words and grunts that don't make any sense. Talk, sing, cry, shout, mumble, whisper! Express whatever needs to be expressed and throw everything out!

b. Allow your arms and body to lose control with your sounds to totally release your energy. Flop over, flap, kick, punch!

c. Do this for 30 seconds without stopping.

d. Rest your hands on your knees.

e. Breathe and calm down. In the stillness and silence, feel how the catharsis - the "letting go" - has penetrated your whole body, from head to toe.

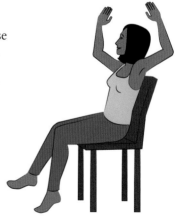

53

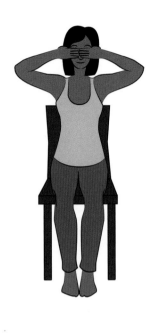

2. BEE'S BREATH

Like you reboot your computer for better for performance, Bee's Breath serves to reboot your mind. It is one of the best breathing exercises to do when you're feeling agitated, frustrated or angry, or you have a headache.

a. Sit tall.

b. Place your thumbs on the cartilage between your cheek and ear - the little flap that mutes your hearing when you press on it (not *in* your ear).

c. Put your other fingers over your eyes, with your elbows out to the side.

d. Take a deep breath and hum out a "bee buzzing" sound with your mouth closed. The sound should come from the bottom of your throat.

e. Focus on the center of your forehead to open up your "Third Eye" and feel the buzzing vibration inside your entire head.

f. Let out all your breath, then breathe in through your nose.

g. Do this 5 times.

h. Breathe and relax with your eyes closed. Feel the calming "buzzing" sensation radiate through your body and mind.

Negative feelings are a part of life. It's how you deal with them that counts. You have complete control over misery! Laugh at it! Throw wild gibberish at it! You'll never look at life the same way again!

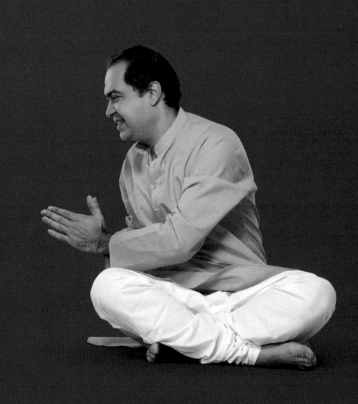

OPENING BELL

BELL

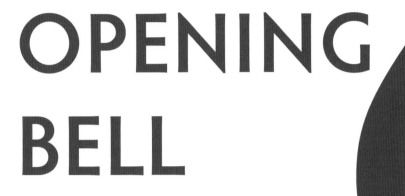

Wake up to Wall Street Yoga

"When you practice yoga with *right* intentions,
it doesn't matter what side of the bed you wake up on."

- GuruNanda

THE NEW YORK STOCK EXCHANGE OPENING BELL MARKS THE BEGINNING OF EACH TRADING DAY.

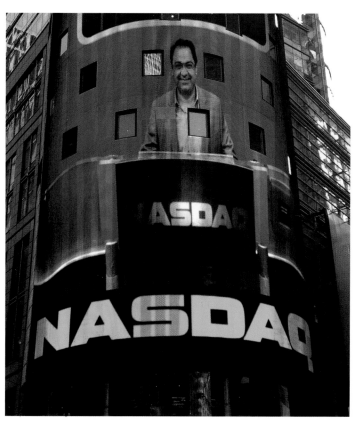

I am proud to say that I had the opportunity to ring that bell. It definitely sets the tone for a day filled with high-octane energy, action… and lots of stress. There is nothing calm about the floor of the New York Stock Exchange. And at the time that I rang the bell, there was nothing calm about *me*. The morning I rang it, I was jet-lagged and sleep-deprived from flying in on the red eye across the country. I ate a room service breakfast of eggs, bacon and toast with butter, plus some cereal. I downed a giant latte with three sugars, and nowater. Needless to say, I had not exercised… in months.

In the stock market, every day is filled with potential. You might have profits. You might have losses. That is a metaphor for life. But it's how you dealwith each circumstance that informs your existence as a whole. Starting your day with a brightness, lightness and optimism sets the tone. However, that doesn't mean you should have expectations about outcomes. It just means to be open to infinite possibilities.

Your Morning Bell Yoga includes simple poses specifically to help you jumpstart your circulation, increase your flexibility and improve your strength. You are getting your mind aware and stable for the hectic day ahead. Your spine will be bolstered to deal with the world outside home.

Although this book gives you yoga routines for various issues and problems, your first 2-minute mantra-based meditation should be done when you wake up. Meditation masters have always believed that morning is the best time to meditate.

SECRETS OF THE SUNRISE

1. **Your brain is quiet** - When you wake up, brain traffic hasn't yet rolled in. Even though thoughts will start up, you're going to benefit from beginning at that peaceful morning place inside.

2. **The WORLD is quiet** - Since everyone is asleep or just waking up, you can enjoy the stillness around you. There aren't the usual distractions, and you can focus on your mantra. This is especially important for beginners. Once you regularly meditate, you can close your eyes anywhere and immediately open the doors to bliss.

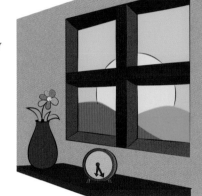

3. **You'll find your focus** - It's good to focus your awareness in the morning before you do anything else. You are going to be downloading information, strategizing and making choices all day. Zero in now before the attention scatter hits. This is like starting the day with a clean desk, instead of a chaotic and cluttered one.

4. **Positivity prevails** - By looking at the day's potential, you can begin with an optimistic, open mind. Remember, leave desire out of the picture and don't worry about results. Meditation will connect your body, mind and spirit, so that you can have a grounded attitude.

Morning Bell Yoga should be done right when you wake up. Use the restroom and brush your teeth. I recommend scraping your tongue with a tongue cleaner. Yogis have been scraping their tongues for hundreds of years. It not only reduces halitosis-breeding bacteria, it activates the salivary glands that aid digestion and it revitalizes the throat.

Morning Bell Yoga should also be done *before* your breakfast or first cup of coffee. After a few days of this **12-MINUTE ROUTINE** (2 minutes of meditation and 10 minutes of poses), you might find that you won't even need the a.m. caffeine boost anymore!

SAY NO TO JOE

Avoid coffee first thing in the morning. Caffeine "stresses" your body, which can slow your digestion. Your digestive fuel tank is empty after a night of sleep, so **EAT WITHIN AN HOUR OF WAKING UP.**

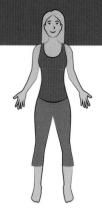

STAND. In yoga, basic standing position is called **MOUNTAIN POSE.** Your feet are parallel, hip distance apart. Your arms are relaxed by your sides. Most importantly, you are standing firmly on the earth, proud and tall like a mountain.

SIT ON A MAT OR BLANKET on the floor in a cross-legged position. Rest your hands on your knees, palms up. Your spine should be straight. Start with your 2-minute mantra-based meditation. Follow the steps in Chapter 4.

1. YOGIC JOGGING

This will get your heart pumping and your blood moving. Remember to try and control your breath. Don't pant. Instead, **breathe**.

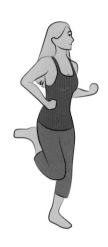

a. Jog in place using both legs. Bring your knees up as high as you comfortably can. Circle your arms gently by your sides. Do 50 jogs.

b. Do 50 more jogs, kicking your feet toward your bottom.

c. Stand in Mountain Pose.

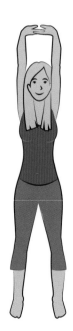

2. PALM TREE POSE

With each deep breath in this polar direction pose, you can actually feel prana (oxygen and nutrients) move into the stretched cell structure, helping to push out toxins and promote cellular regeneration.

a. Stand tall in Mountain Pose and lift your arms in the air.

b. Interlock your fingers and turn your hands so your palms face

upward. Lift your heels. Focus on a fixed object in front of you to maintain your balance.

c. Feel the pull upwards while your toes press into the floor. Remember to keep your shoulders relaxed - don't hunch them up by your ears.

d. Take 5 deep breaths all the way down to your navel.

e. Gently lower your heels, release your arms to your sides and stand in Mountain Pose.

3. SWAYING PALM TREE POSE

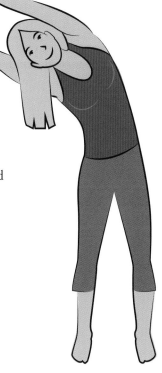

a. Standing in Mountain Pose, interlock your fingers with your index fingers pointing up, and raise your arms.

a. Ground yourself into the floor while distributing weight equally between your feet.

b. Keep your hips forward and bend at the waist to your right. Take 5 deep breaths. Feel the stretch on the side of your torso, but don't let your hips lose their straight alignment.

c. Bend at the waist to your left and take 5 deep breaths.

d. Do the right and left side again, extending a little further with each exhalation.

e. Return to Mountain Pose.

4. FORWARD FOLD POSE

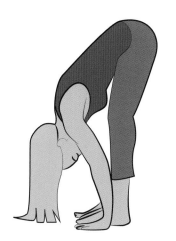

a. Start in Mountain Pose. Inhale and reach your arms up. They should be parallel.

b. Exhale as you slowly fold your upper body from the hips and try to touch your toes. If you feel inflexible, bend your knees slightly. You'll experience a gentle stretch in your hamstrings.

c. Let your head, upper body and hands hang loosely.

d. Take 10 deep breaths. With every exhale, try and touch your fingers to your toes.

e. Roll your body up one vertebrae at a time and stand in Mountain Pose.

5. CHAIR POSE

a. From Mountain Pose, inhale and raise your arms straight up next to your ears.

b. Exhale and bend your knees as if you are sitting in a chair. Try and get your thighs parallel to the floor with your bottom pushed out.

c. Lift your heart as you breathe, bringing your hips even lower. (though never *below* your knees). Keep your arms straight up. If you need "training wheels," hold onto the back of a chair for balance.

d. Take 5 deep breaths.

e. Inhale with a higher lift of the arms and stand in Mountain Pose, bringing your arms down.

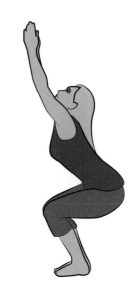

6. SHOULDER ROLLS

A heart-opener.

a. Standing in Mountain Pose, bend your arms and bring your hands to your shoulders.

b. Make full, slow circle rotations, keeping your fingers at your shoulders. These circles should be as big as possible. Do 10 forward.

c. Do 10 backwards.

d. Return to Mountain Pose.

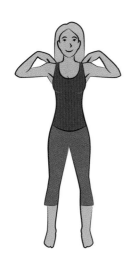

7. ARM-OUTS

The natural fight against gravity during this exercise will promote strong arms and toned shoulders.

a. Remain in Mountain Pose. Lift your arms straight out to the sides and make tight fists. Circle your arms 20 times clockwise, then 20 times counter-clockwise.

b. Keep your arms straight out and flex your wrists up and down 20 times.

c. Keep your arms straight out and circle your hands at the wrist. Do 10 circles each direction.

d. Release your arms to your sides and stand in Mountain Pose.

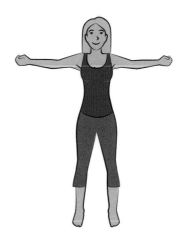

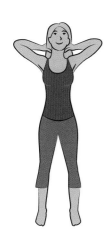

8. HEAD PRESS

Strengthens neck muscles, alleviates bone pressure and reduces C-spine pain.

a. Start in Mountain Pose. Put your hands behind your head with your palms facing you.

b. Press your head back against your hands. Keep your head straight.

c. Take 5 deep breaths.

d. Press your right palm against the right side of your head. Keep your head straight.

e. Take 5 deep breaths.

f. Press the left palm against the left side of your head. Keep your head straight.

g. Take 5 deep breaths.

h. Press both palms against your forehead. Keep your head straight.

i. Take 5 deep breaths.

9. NECK STRETCHES

"Pre-stretch" the muscles that tend to get tighter as the day goes on.

a. From Mountain Pose, bend your head to the right, then the left. Do this slowly with 1 deep breath for each side.

b. Repeat 5 times each side. Every time, you should be able to take your head further.

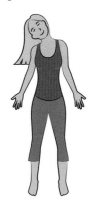

10. LUNGE TWIST

Twists are great toxin eliminators.

a. From Mountain Pose, lunge forward with your right foot.

b. Put your palms together in Prayer Position, elbows out to the sides.

c. Twist your upper body to the right and place your left elbow on your right knee.

d. Take 5 deep breaths.

e. Repeat on the left side.

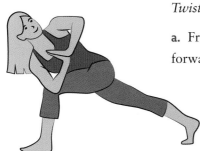

CORPSE POSE

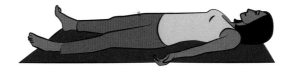

BONUS POSES:

1. SUN SALUTATION

Considered the Mother of all asanas, the Sun Salutation is designed to revive and energize your mind, body and spirit because it includes almost every element of a full practice: breath, stretching and strength. On days when I'm too busy to squeeze in even 10 minutes of yoga, I do 10 Sun Salutations. Then, I'm refreshed and ready to go.

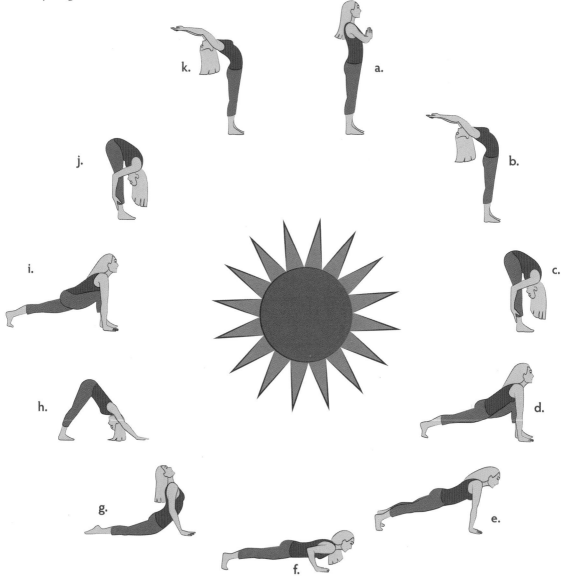

A simple rule for **breathing** *during this exercise:* **breathe out** *as you move gratefully toward Mother Earth,* **breath in** *as your raise yourself to stand tall against the pressures of life. This "in and out" is important for balancing ego, work, and life in general.*

a. Stand in Mountain Pose with your palms together in Prayer Position, thumbs touching your heart.

b. Inhale and reach your arms up and slightly back. Gaze toward the sky, feeling a long stretch from neck to feet.

c. Exhale and fold forward from your hips. Touch your hands to the floor. Bend your knees slightly if you feel inflexible.

d. With your hands on the floor, inhale and extend your right leg back in a lunge. You can put your knee down or keep it lifted.

e. Bring your left foot back and exhale, lowering your knees and calves to the floor.

f. With an inhale, press your palms into the floor and straighten your arms to push your torso up. Gaze up. **This is Cobra Pose.**

g. Exhale and lift your bottom to the sky. Straighten your legs. You

will be in an inverted "V" position. **This is Downward-Facing Dog Pose.**

h. Inhale and bring your right foot forward, back into a lunge.

i. Exhale and bring your left foot to meet your right in a Forward Fold.

j. Inhale and roll your upper body up to standing.

k. Exhale in Mountain Pose, hands to Prayer Position.

For 10 Sun Salutations, do 5 with the right leg first, then 5 with the left.

2. BALANCING TREE POSE

a. Stand in Mountain Pose.

b. Balance on the right leg and bend the left leg, turning the left knee out.

c. Place the sole of the left foot on the right calf or thigh. (Do not place the sole of the foot on the knee. This can produce a knee injury).

d. Balance with your arms down or in the air. If your arms are in the air, you can place your palms together with your fingers pointed up.

e. Focus your eyes on one point to help you balance.

f. Take 5 deep breaths.

g. Do the opposite side.

h. Return to Mountain Pose with your hands in Prayer Position and take 1 deep breath.

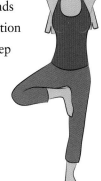

LAUGHTER YOGA (Chapter 5) is also a fantastic way to start your day.

Whether you wake up to the sun shining or to stormy skies, your mind, body and spirit will be ready to take on the day when you do a little Wall Street Yoga. Ring your own "opening bell" and set the tone for your life.

BALANCE YOUR PORTFOLIO

Yoga for Weight Loss and Management

"A man is the sum of the food he puts in his body
plus the thoughts that occur in his mind."

- GuruNanda

RECENTLY, I WAS WATCHING AN INFOMERCIAL FOR A DIET PRODUCT

in which a smorgasbord of food was literally sitting in a disgusting animated globule of oil. Instead of ingesting a pill, why not just avoid those foods and that globule in the first place? This made me think of P.U.R.E.: Perspiration, Urination, Respiration, Excretion. That's how the body cleans itself of toxins. But how do toxins get produced? We've already talked about stress. There are also outside forces, like pollution, GMO's, medications, etc. A large bulk of toxins are produced from undigested food because, most simply, we eat too much. We're a society of excess.

When a child is born, a parent's "duty" is to feed him a balanced diet, complete with the right amount of ingredients, vitamins, minerals, fats, protein and carbohydrates. However, although my own mom constantly told me to "Eat this, eat that, drink this, drink that," I still ate what tasted and felt good to me. Children start out approaching food in a very instinctual way. But as time went on, that "eating intuition" vanished. I ate due to parental and peer pressure, and later, because of stress, depression, habit and time restrictions (fast food!).

After I'd go out to eat with friends, I would come home "hungry." I got into the habit of opening the refrigerator to find a sweet treat or something to munch on. It was my *mind* that was not satisfied, though I could feel my belly bulging. Combine my eating habits with my sedentary desktop lifestyle, and I ballooned to 186 pounds. I honestly didn't even know what tasted good anymore. When we eat in excess, our bodies don't know how to get rid of so many toxins. We're not perspiring or breathing properly because we're sitting at our desks or in our cars. Our lymphatic system literally chokes on the overflow of toxins and sends these toxins to the main storage areas - fat cells. In 2000, everyone put money in technology stocks, and the market crashed. The best investment advice has always been to balance your portfolio. The same can be said for our eating habits. As long as you listen to yourself, you will start to eat right and in moderation.

After I talk to others about my weight loss, some people decide to restrict their food, trying to live on broccoli and boiled chicken, even at fine restaurants and family gatherings. But my advice is moderation. It's okay to eat whatever you want periodically. Be gentle with yourself. If you're too strict, you'll be quicker to give up your new eating plan altogether. This is not a week - or even a month - diet program. It's a lifelong journey, so relax, breathe and embark on the right nutritional direction slowly.

Wall Street Yoga is not a diet program. It is a lifestyle that centers on balance, the focus of Ayurveda. The word "Ayurveda" in Sanskrit means "Knowledge of Life." Ayurveda provides both curative and preventive measures for optimal physical, emotional and spiritual well-being.

AYURVEDA PHILOSOPHY
Balance = Health
Imbalance = Disease

When you attain balance, you will attain your ideal weight.

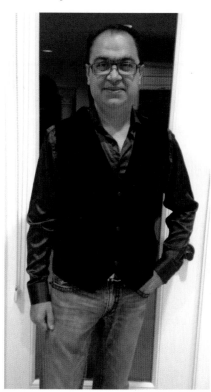

In my yogic studies, I learned about eating everything that has PRANIC VALUE, not caloric value. These are foods that possess "life force." They are the elements of what I call "Happy Eating." The foods that make your ATMAN (in Hindu, the essence of a person) happy are the foods that have high pranic value. Again, moderation is key.

What are foods with pranic value?

- Foods made with love, because you remember how your mother, father or grandparent cooked your favorite dishes. Einstein said, "Energy cannot be created or destroyed, it can only be changed from one form to another." The same applies to cooking. Feelings of love are transferred to these special dishes and converted to pranic value.

- Live foods like sprouted grains, beans, vegetables, nuts, seeds, etc. These assist with digestion and the assimilation of nutrients.

- Foods with vivid colors and fragrant scents.

Eating while working, watching TV, driving your car or talking on the phone sucks the pranic value out of your food. Eating with awareness makes food taste better. More digestive juices and enzymes act on every morsel, arousing your taste buds and making your atman happy.

PROCESSED SUGAR HAS ZERO PRANIC VALUE. Though some natural sugar is okay in moderation, sodas, cookies, candy and the like are addictive and harmful. The imbalance in the body caused by excessive processed sugar intake manifests in symptoms such as fatigue, irritability, skin problems, on-going pain, constipation, diarrhea, weight gain, depression and high blood pressure. If you are going to consume sugar, it should be in the purest form from foods like raw fruits.

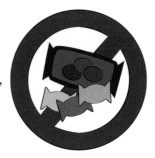

10 HAPPY EATING "RULES"

1. Eat at least 50% natural fresh, seasonal and regional fruits and vegetables. Avoid canned, processed, preserved and fast foods. Stay close to what your ancestors ate. Always ask yourself, "Am I eating food made by nature or a factory?" If your answer is the latter, then find a healthier option.

2. Snack minimally between meals. Snacking disturbs food digestion, which takes up to four hours. Make any snacks small, like a handful of nuts or a gluten-free cookie or cracker. After I cut out wheat and gluten for 30 days, I felt better overall and it's been easy to keep them out of my diet.

3. Eat lightest in the evening.

4. Avoid coffee first thing in the morning. Caffeine "stresses" your body, which can slow your digestion. Your digestive fuel tank is empty after a night of sleep, so give it food within an hour of waking up (but *after* your Mourning Yoga routine, if you choose to do it).

5. Sip your beverages. Don't gulp. Drink 100 ml. of water every 30 minutes during the day - sip by sip.

6. Avoid dairy as much as possible. The human digestive system is not designed to absorb milk products. Try soy and almond alternatives.

7. Cut out sugar that doesn't come from natural sources like fruit.

8. Have a teaspoon of ginger juice with every meal. In Ayurveda, it boosts your "digestive fire." Plus, it's shown to be an antioxidant.

9. Never stand while eating. Sit at a table (not your desk) and treat yourself to a nice meal as if you are in a restaurant. Close your laptop and put away your cellphone. Phone calls, texts and emails take a bite out of your true enjoyment.

10. EAT SLOWLY! You will benefit from maximum nutrients. When your food pre-digests with the enzymes in saliva as you chew, your body will appropriately signal "full."

As an inventor and a perpetual science "student," I am a firm supporter of modern medicine. Modern medicine - from antibiotics to surgery to imaging, plus assured balanced nutrition due to irrigation and agricultural advancement - has helped increase our average life span from 40 to 80 years. However, new complex-lifestyle diseases like diabetes, hypertension, heart disease, stroke and cancer, have been growing. And stress plays a big part in this pandemic. Consequently, the medical industry is progressively accepting the importance of integrating mind-body practices with Western methodologies, and doctors are increasingly recommending yoga.

AN "APERITIF" ASANA: HERO'S POSE

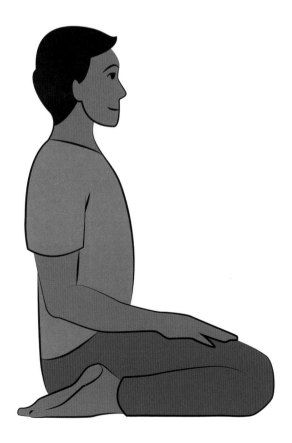

HERO'S POSE

Do this pose after every meal to help direct all the blood to the stomach and promote better digestion.

a. Sit on your knees.

b. Put your palms on your thighs.

c. When you become more flexible, you can slide your bottom to the floor.

d. Take 5 deep breaths.

FACT: No food of plant origin contains any cholesterol!

THE DOWNLOW ON H20:

My good friend was forcefully gulping from a 32-oz. water bottle. He said he thought he *needed* to drink 2 liters a day, because that's what we're told by fitness and diet experts. In reality, too much water at one time causes electrolyte imbalance, because our kidneys can't flush fast enough. It's better to drink water in smaller amounts several times a day.

Guess what? I'm a foodie. I love to eat! But I've learned a system of "accounts and balances." If I eat more one day, I will eat less the next. I even drink alcohol – *in moderation*. So what's a typical daily menu like for me?

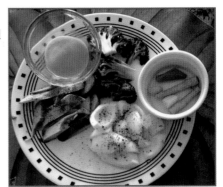

BREAKFAST - This will not seem like a traditional breakfast, but it is a far healthier choice than the omelets, toast and cereal I wolfed down 40 pounds ago. Again, according to Ayurveda, breakfast should be consumed within one hour of waking up.

- 1 tsp. ginger juice, 1 tsp. of apple cider vinegar, and a little fruit juice to mask the taste.

- 2 pieces each of boiled garlic, ginger, amla (Indian gooseberry) and turmeric. When garlic is boiled, it will not make your breath stink.

- 3 scrambled egg whites (vegetarians can use soy egg substitute)

- Fresh greens, lightly sautéed (broccoli, spinach, kale or chard)

- 1 avocado, sliced (avocados are *good* fat)

An alternative to this is to have a mono-fruit breakfast (one type of fruit only). Morning is the best time to eat fruit. When the stomach and intestines are empty, the body can extract the natural energy from the fruits easily and provide energy to start the day.

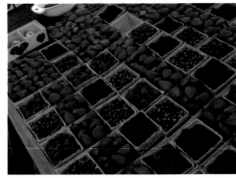

SNACK

- ½ cup of raw, unsalted nuts

LUNCH - The "digestive fire" is at its peak at midday. The best time to have a hearty meal is between 11 a.m. to 1 p.m. Lunch feeds the body enough nutrition for the day, so you won't crave a heavy meal later in the evening.

- Grilled or baked fish or chicken. Lentils are a good protein alternative for vegetarians.
- Brown rice
- Salad

SNACK

- 1 gluten-free cookie or a handful of nuts
- Tea

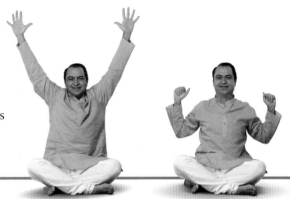

YOGI COFFEE

The afternoon is prime time for Yogi Coffee! You don't need to wait in line or pay $4.50. It's free and you can do it anywhere. When you're done, you'll have a delightfully lightheaded, caffeinated feeling.

1. Sit in a cross-legged position on the floor or in a basic seated position in a chair.
2. Swiftly move your arms up and down.
3. Breathe through your *nose only*. Inhale as your arms go up. Exhale as your arms come down. Your breaths are swift during this exercise.
4. Do 50 repetitions. 1 is up, 2 is down, 3 is up...

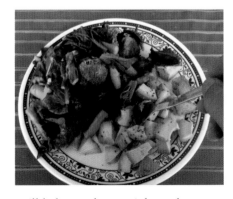

DINNER - Eat a light dinner consisting of easy-to-digest foods between 5 - 6 p.m.

- 2 vegetables, boiled
- A small piece of chicken or fish. I try to avoid meats because they take longer to digest.
- Or, to go super light while still getting protein, eat boiled edamame as a main course.

Asanas will support this healthy way of eating. The combination will help you lose weight and *maintain* that ideal weight for the long haul.

"HAPPY WEIGHT" ROUTINE

The following asanas help promote weight loss. Do not do them directly before or after a meal, but at some point during the day if you are trying to trim pounds. **START THIS ROUTINE IN A SEATED CROSS-LEGGED POSITION WITH YOUR SPINE STRAIGHT.**

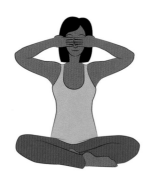

1. BEE'S BREATH

This pose will help stop erratic eating behavior.

a. Sit tall. Place your thumbs on the cartilage between your cheek and ear - the little flap that mutes your hearing when you press on it (not *in* your ear).

b. Put your other fingers over your eyes with your elbows out to the sides.

c. Take a deep breath and hum out a "bee buzzing" sound with your mouth closed. The sound should come from the bottom of your throat.

d. Focus on the center of your forehead to open up your "Third Eye" and feel the buzzing vibration inside your entire head.

e. Through your nose, let out all your breath, then breathe in.

f. Do this 5 times.

g. Breathe and relax with your eyes closed. Feel the calming "buzzing" sensation radiate through your body and mind.

2. KAPALABHATI BREATHING

Expels toxic gases and activates the diaphragm.

a. Remain seated. Through your *nose only*, take a deep breath and exhale quickly, making a "puff out" sound.

b. Focus on a forceful exhale, not on the inhale. Your chest will rise with every exhale.

c. Perform 20 breaths.

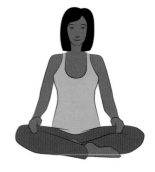

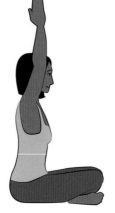

3. BELLOW'S BREATH

Flood your lungs with oxygen. If you have high blood pressure, do this exercise with your arms relaxed on your thighs. Breathe gently.

a. In your seated position, press your arms up with a swift inhale through your *nose only*.

b. Pull your arms down with a swift exhale through your *nose only*.

c. Your chest will puff out when you inhale, retract when you exhale.

d. Repeat 10 times.

e. Relax your arms and take a deep breath.

4. FIRE'S BREATH

Increases metabolism to help you burn calories more efficiently.

a. Make sure you are still sitting with your spine straight. Take a deep breath in for 5 counts, through your *nose only*. Feel the inhale deep in your stomach. Simultaneously, pull your stomach up toward the ribs, so it will look hollowed out.

b. Exhale through your nose and release your stomach.

c. Repeat once more.

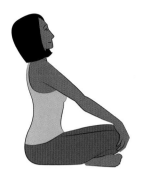

5. PALM TREE POSE

a. Stand tall in Mountain Pose with your feet parallel, hip distance apart. Lift your arms in the air.

b. Interlock your fingers and turn your hands so your palms face upward.

c. Lift your heels. Focus on a fixed object in front of you to maintain your balance.

d. Feel the pull upwards while your toes press into the floor. Remember to keep your shoulders relaxed - don't hunch them up by your ears.

e. Take 5 deep breaths all the way down to your navel.

f. Gently lower your heels, release your arms to your sides and stand in Mountain Pose.

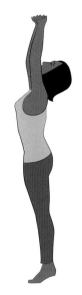

6. SWAYING PALM TREE POSE

a. Interlock your fingers with your index fingers pointed up and raise your arms.

b. Ground yourself into the floor while distributing weight equally between your feet.

c. Keep your hips forward and bend at the waist to your right. Take 5 deep breaths. Feel the stretch on the side of your torso, but don't let your hips lose their straight alignment.

d. Bend at the waist to your left and take 5 deep breaths.

e. Do the right and left side again, extending a little further with each exhalation.

f. Return to Mountain Pose.

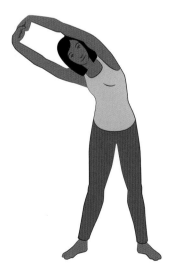

7. CHILD'S POSE

a. Sit on your knees and reach your arms out in front of you, folding your torso over your thighs. Keep your bottom down.

b. With flat palms, spread your fingers wide. Your face should be close to the floor.

c. Take 5 deep breaths.

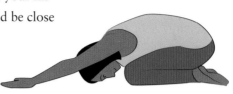

8. CAT-COW POSE

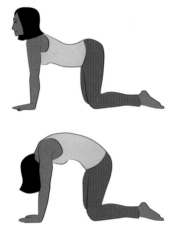

a. On your hands and knees, lift your belly button gently toward your spine to make your back flat. Your neck should be long and the top of your head forward.

b. Simultaneously, lift your head up and your bottom up, curving your back in a slight "U" shape.

c. Take 5 deep breaths.

d. Round your spine in an upside-down "U" shape.

e. Drop your head and gaze at your navel.

f. Take 5 deep breaths.

g. Do each pose once more.

h. Come back to neutral position with your back flat and the top of your head forward.

9. FROG POSE (TRADITIONAL INDIAN VERSION)

a. Sit on your knees.

b. Make fists and bring them together so that your thumbs touch your navel. Your elbows will be out to the sides.

c. Exhale and lean forward over your fists. Try to touch your chest to your knees.

d. Take 5 deep breaths.

e. Sit up and relax.

f. Repeat once more.

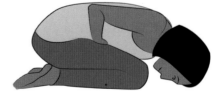

10. COBRA POSE

a. Lie on your stomach with your toes pointed.

b. Place your hands underneath your chest, palms down.

c. Press down to lift your torso up. Gaze up.

d. Take 5 deep breaths.

e. Release your torso down and relax.

f. Repeat once more.

BONUS POSES:

1. BOAT POSE

This is a fantastic ab-flattener.

a. Sit with your knees bent.

b. Keep your abs firm and lift your legs.

c. Straighten your legs.

d. Reach your arms past your knees. If you need help balancing, lightly hold on to your thighs.

e. Take 5 deep breaths.

f. Bend your knees and put your feet back on the floor.

g. Lay back and relax.

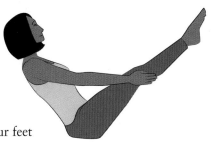

2. WARRIOR 1 POSE

a. Stand tall in Mountain Pose, then step your feet wide apart.

b. With your hands on your hips, turn your right leg and foot out 90 degrees while you turn your left leg and foot in 45 degrees.

c. Square your chest in the direction of your right leg.

d. Inhale and lift your arms above your head. Bring your palms together.

e. Exhale and bend your right knee to a 90-degree angle.

f. Take 5 deep breaths.

g. Straighten your right leg and return to Mountain Pose.

h. Repeat on the other side.

i. Take 5 deep breaths.

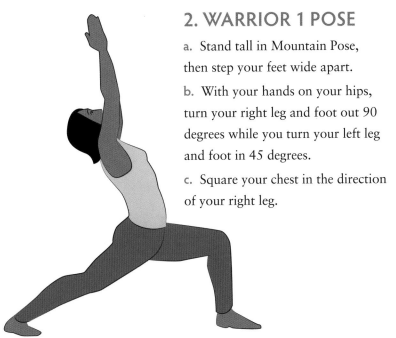

The first person I ever inspired to do yoga after my transformation was my younger brother, Sumit. He now sits on the International World Ayurveda Council Board.

SUMIT'S STORY

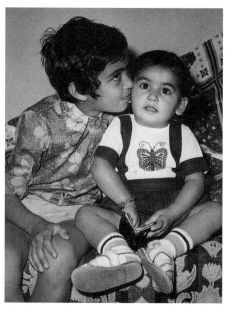

I was not a believer. Even though yoga is as ancient as my culture, I did not practice. I didn't meditate.
I was a firm supporter of modern medicine.

I had just turned 40 and thought that my lifestyle was just fine. I exercised for an hour or more a day. I ate dinner early. I followed the recommendations of my doctors. Still, I had high blood pressure and high cholesterol, and I would fall sick with cold and cough every two months. I had a history of migraines, but the frequency was increasing to two to three a week. I was always tired, yet I could not sleep because my mind was restless. Then, my dad had a renal transplant. His kidneys failed and he had to go through
multiple hospitalizations. At the hospital with my dad, I thought to myself, "Here is where I will end up
if I don't change."

My brother introduced me to Ayurveda and yoga. I gave up packaged foods, fast foods, sodas and anything processed or made in a factory. I drink plenty of water to ensure I'm properly hydrated.

I lost over 20 pounds. My migraines disappeared, as did the colds and flus. My blood pressure stabilized and my cholesterol lowered. Most importantly, my self-esteem rose. People tell me that I don't look my age. That's probably because I feel much younger than
I am.

Here is what I've learned that continues to change my life for the better:

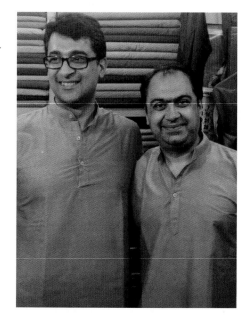

- Eat your food like water and drink your water like food. This is all about eating slow, because when you chew well, your food liquefies and mixes with your saliva, which is key to proper digestion.

- Rather than look at our mental, emotional and physical health problems in a holistic manner, we tend to just treat the symptoms associated with these issues, not the underlying cause. As one problem is treated, another one appears because the body is trying to communicate the real problem at hand. The cycle continues until the root cause is finally uncovered, usually after we've been diagnosed with a chronic illness. we've been diagnosed with a chronic illness.

- Fasting is one of the most effective detoxification methods, and has been shown to help build our immune system. One day of complete fast a week (or only fruit) is very effective in cleaning up our digestive system. (Author's note: Remember, neither Sumit or I are doctors. Check with your doctor before you change your diet or fast.)

- There are three factors that are very important for a healthy life: good nutrition, sleep and exercise. A good rest is the body's time to repair and renew the cells. Our body has an amazing ability to renew itself.

You have only one body to live in. If you don't take care of it, where will you live?
- Sumit Nanda

Our modern day lifestyle has become increasingly "artificial." We are living in man-made cities. Foods are genetically modified to increase production. They are laced with pesticides. Animal products are full of growth hormones and antibiotics. We are breathing pollution from all of the emissions coming from factories and engines. We are drinking water treated with chlorine and fluoride, using cosmetics and deodorants to look and smell good, and on top of all, we are increasingly using drugs and medicines to curb symptoms when our bodies are really trying to tell us to *get our house in order*. Happy Eating focuses on getting back to nature and an instinctual way of nourishing our bodies.

After I lost weight, a woman asked me if the results were long-term or short-term. In turn, I asked her, "If you wash your clothes tonight and wear them tomorrow, do you expect them to remain clean long-term? You have to continue washing your clothes to keep them fresh." Healthy weight maintenance takes a conscious effort. Eating right doesn't need to be difficult, but it must be consistent.

Worship your body and you will discover it will bring you much joy.

THE RUBBER BAND EFFECT

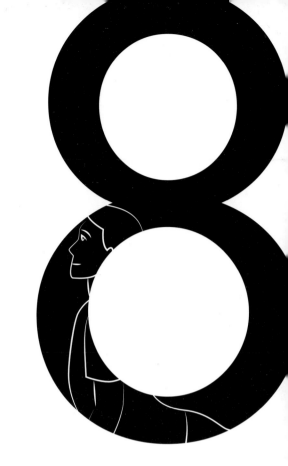

Yoga for Back Pain and Sciatica

"Type A personalities carry the weight of the world on their backs."

- GuruNanda

BACK PAIN HAS BEEN SHOWN TO PLAGUE OVER 27,000 U.S. ADULTS

a year. It should be no surprise that the annual cost of chronic pain in the U.S., including health care and expenses, and lost productivity, is estimated at $560-635 billion, according to a 2011 report released by the Institute of Medicine. In 2011, 219 million opioid prescriptions were sold by pharmacies, up from 180 million in 2006. Opioids, like Vicodin, are highly addictive painkillers. Due to chronic back pain, I was a pain meds addict... until I started doing yoga.

Back pain can be caused by muscle or ligament strain, or by a bulging or ruptured disk. If you pick up heavy weight and your muscles are not strong enough, then all the load goes to the vertebrae, causing a rupture in the disk. Excess body weight, inactivity, arthritis, osteoporosis, bad posture, scoliosis, and poor alignment of vertebrae and ribs can also lead to back pain.

Studies show we spend an average of 7.7 hours a day sitting. In America, many occupations require long hours behind a desk. The spine is designed to hold loads in its neutral S-curved position, which naturally adopts when you stand up. But the seated position alters those curves. This creates lower back pain, and, according to a 2010 Global Burden of Disease study, lower back pain is the leading cause of disability across the world.

The majority of all physical ailments have a psychological component.
STORED EMOTIONS EXACERBATE BACK PAIN.

After a large sell-off in the stock market, there is a tendency for the market to bounce back right away. That's called **THE RUBBER BAND EFFECT**. Similarly, when you learn to "sell off" your stress by letting go of control, expectations and the desire for a particular outcome, your body, mind and spirit will find new flexibility and strength... like a rubber band.

Most people actually relate yoga to stretching. Images that come into mind are people twisting themselves into knots and doing back bends like circus acrobats. However, the poses must be done with conscious effort and care to get the most out of them and to avoid injury. **Doing the poses correctly, with proper alignment, is THE NUMBER ONE MOST IMPORTANT FACTOR.** Even after practicing for so many years, I am unable to do some complicated poses. That's fine! Every *body* has its limitations. Respect yours. By breathing through the movements, you will be able to "open" up your body and reap the ultimate benefits.

My best friend, an orthopedic surgeon, often tells me that yoga may put him and his colleagues out of business. The stronger the muscle around the vertebrae, the less pain. Yoga poses increase muscle strength and core stability to support the spine.

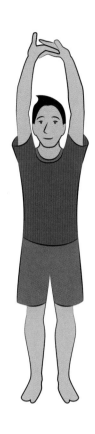

1. PALM TREE POSE

a. Stand tall in Mountain Pose with your feet parallel, hip distance apart. Lift your arms in the air.

b. Interlock your fingers and turn your hands so your palms face upward.

c. Lift your heels. Focus on a fixed object in front of you to maintain your balance.

d. Feel the pull upwards while your toes press into the floor. Remember to keep your shoulders relaxed - don't hunch them up by your ears.

e. Take 5 deep breaths all the way down to your navel.

f. Gently lower your heels, release your arms to your sides and stand in Mountain Pose.

2. SWAYING PALM TREE POSE

a. Interlock your fingers with your index fingers pointed up and raise your arms.

b. Ground yourself into the floor while distributing weight equally between your feet.

c. Keep your hips forward and bend at the waist to your right. Take 5 deep breaths. Feel the stretch on the side of your torso, but don't let your hips lose their straight alignment.

d. Bend at the waist to your left and take 5 deep breaths.

e. Do the right and left side again, extending a little further with each exhalation.

f. Return to Mountain Pose.

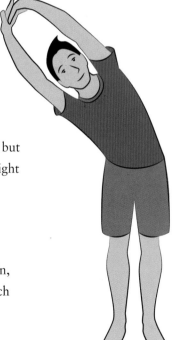

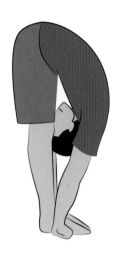

3. FORWARD FOLD WITH FISTS

The fists in this pose use the healing magic of gravity to make space between your spinal bones.

a. From Mountain Pose, fold forward from the hips.

b. Try to keep your legs straight. If you feel inflexible, bend your knees slightly.

c. Bend your elbows out to the sides, laying one forearm on top of the other.

d. Make fists and squeeze them.

e. Take 10 deep breaths.

f. Release your hands and arms and let them hang to the floor.

g. Roll up with a round back and stand in Mountain Pose.

4. CAT-COW POSE

a. On your hands and knees, gently lift your belly button toward your spine to make your back flat. Your neck should be long and the top of your head forward.

b. Simultaneously, lift your head up and your bottom up, curving your back in a slight "U" shape.

c. Take 5 deep breaths.

d. Round your spine in an upside-down "U" shape.

e. Drop your head and gaze at your navel.

f. Take 5 deep breaths.

g. Do each pose once more.

h. Come back to neutral position with your back flat and the top of your head forward.

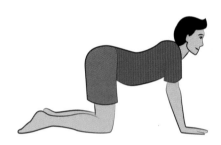

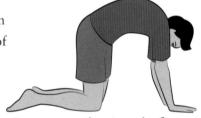

5. KING PIGEON POSE

This is a great hip-opener.

a. Start on your hands and knees.

b. Slide your right knee forward toward your left hand and lay it down so your knee is facing out. Your foot should be underneath your chest.

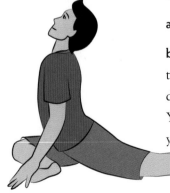

c. Press your palms into the floor and your arms straight. Your chest should be forward, along with your head.

d. Take 5 deep breaths.

e. Move back to your hands and knees.

f. Do the other side.

g. Take 5 deep breaths.

6. CHILD'S POSE

a. Sit on your knees and reach your arms out in front of you, folding your torso over your thighs. Keep your bottom down.

b. With flat palms, spread your fingers wide. Your face should be close to the floor.

c. Take 5 deep breaths.

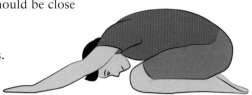

7. DOWNWARD-FACING DOG POSE

a. Start on your hands and knees.

b. Push down on your hands and lift your bottom up to the sky, straightening your arms and legs. You will be in an inverted "V" position.

c. Take 5 deep breaths.

d. Go back to your hands and knees.

8. ONE-LEGGED SEATED TWIST

a. Sit with your legs out in front of you.

b. Bend your right knee and place your right foot over your straight left leg.

c. Place your elbow on the inside of your bent right leg. Your palm is in a "wave" position. Press your elbow against your knee so you can feel the twist in your waist and back.

d. Take 5 deep breaths.

e. Switch sides.

f. Take 5 deep breaths.

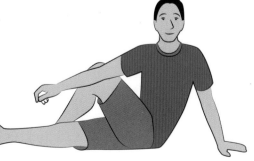

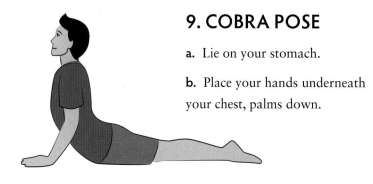

9. COBRA POSE

a. Lie on your stomach.

b. Place your hands underneath your chest, palms down.

c. Press down to lift your torso up. Gaze up.

d. Take 5 deep breaths.

e. Release your torso down and relax.

f. Repeat once more.

10. THREAD THE NEEDLE POSE

Feel the stretch in your shoulders and across your upper back.

a. On your hands and knees, slide the right hand underneath your body and across your chest to the left.

b. Your right shoulder and side of the head should sit comfortably on the floor.

c. Take 5 deep breaths.

d. Switch arms.

e. Take 5 deep breaths.

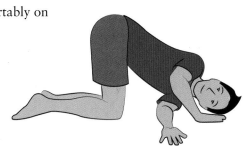

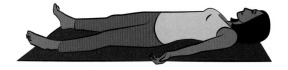

CORPSE POSE

BONUS POSES:

1. FLYING POSE

a. Lie on your stomach.

b. Reach your arms out in front of your head.

c. Keep your legs straight and point your toes.

d. Lift your arms and legs. You might not get far off the ground.

e. Take 5 deep breaths.

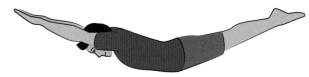

2. WIND REMOVING POSE

a. Lie on your back.

b. Pull your right leg into your chest, bent.

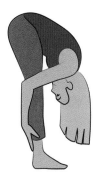

c. Take 5 deep breaths.

d. Release the leg back to the floor, straight.

e. Pull your left leg into your chest, bent.

f. Take 5 deep breaths.

SCIATICA is a specific type of back pain caused by the compression or irritation of one of five spinal nerve roots of each sciatic nerve. It can also be caused by the compression or irritation of the left, right or both sciatic nerves. In addition to lower back pain, sciatica symptoms include:

- Buttock pain and numbness
- Pain or weakness in various parts of the leg and foot
- A "pins-and-needles" sensation or tingling in the leg
- Typically, symptoms only manifest on one side of the body

Practicing yoga can help you heal sciatica, but practicing yoga *wrong* can worsen the condition. **Go into each pose slowly and with breath.**

"RUBBER BAND EFFECT" ROUTINE FOR SCIATICA

1. FORWARD FOLD POSE

a. Stand tall in Mountain Pose with your feet parallel, hip distance apart. Inhale and reach your arms up.

b. Exhale as you slowly fold your upper body from the hips and try to touch your toes. If you feel inflexible, bend your knees slightly. You'll experience a gentle stretch in your hamstrings.

c. Let your head, upper body and hands hang loosely.

d. Take 10 deep breaths. With every exhale, try and touch your fingers to your toes.

e. Roll your body up one vertebrae at a time and stand in Mountain Pose.

2. DOWNWARD-FACING DOG POSE

a. Start on your hands and knees.

b. Push down on your hands and lift your bottom up to the sky, straightening your arms and legs. You will be in an inverted "V" position.

c. Take 5 deep breaths.

d. Go back to your hands and knees.

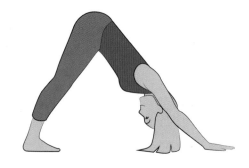

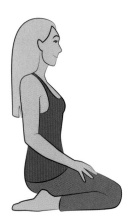

3. HERO'S POSE

a. Sit on your knees.

b. Put your palms on your thighs.

c. When you become more flexible, you can slide your bottom to the floor.

d. Take 5 deep breaths.

4. KING PIGEON POSE

a. Start on your hands and knees.

b. Slide your right knee forward toward your left hand and lay it down so your knee is facing out. Your foot should be underneath your chest.

c. Press your palms into the floor and your arms straight. Your chest should be forward, along with your head.

d. Take 5 deep breaths.

e. Move back to your hands and knees.

f. Do the other side.

g. Take 5 deep breaths.

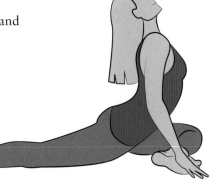

5. COW'S FACE POSE

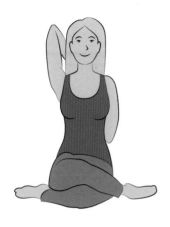

a. Sit with both legs straight out.

b. Bend your right leg in front of you, knee and calf flat on the floor.

c. Lift your left leg, bend your knee, and place your left knee on top of your right knee. Your left calf should be stacked horizontally on top of your right calf. *If someone were looking at you, your legs would look like a cow's mouth!*

d. Reach your right arm up and your left arm down.

e. Reach them behind you and try to clasp your hands. Don't worry if your hands don't reach each other. Just go for the stretch in your shoulders and across your chest.

f. Take 5 deep breaths.

g. Do the same thing with the other leg and the opposite arm position.

h. Take 5 deep breaths.

6. WESTERN'S POSE

a. Sit with your legs straight out in front of you.

b. Reach out and touch your toes. If you feel inflexible at first, bend your knees slightly.

c. Take 10 deep breaths.

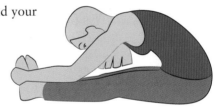

7. RECLINED THIGH OVER THIGH POSE

a. Lie on your back with your legs bent. Put your hands behind your head, elbows out.

b. Cross your right leg over your left.

c. Twist your lower body toward the left. Try and get your crossed legs to touch the floor.

d. Take 5 deep breaths.

e. Cross your left leg over your right.

f. Twist your lower body toward the right.

g. Take 5 deep breaths.

8. SIMPLIFIED PIGEON POSE

a. Remain flat on your back with your knees bent.

b. Turn your right knee out and put your right foot on your left knee.

c. Wrap your hands around your left thigh and gently put your legs toward you.

d. Take 5 deep breaths.

e. Do the same on the opposite side.

e. Take 5 deep breaths.

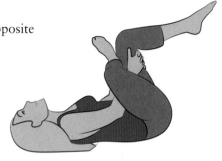

9. YOGIC CYCLING - BENT LEGS

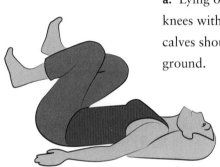

a. Lying on your back, bend your knees with your feet lifted. Your calves should be parallel to the ground.

b. Slowly cycle your legs. Make sure you keep your core tight, pulling your belly button toward the floor. This will ensure your back stays down flat.

c. Cycle 20 times, both legs.

10. YOGIC CYCLING - STRAIGHT LEGS

a. Lying on your back, lift your right leg to a 45-degree angle. Keep it straight, with only a slight bend at the knee, and point your toes.

b. Circle your leg 10 times one direction, then 10 times the other direction.

c. Do the same cycling with the left leg at a 45-degree angle. Remember to keep your core tight and your back flat.

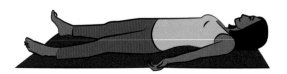

CORPSE POSE

BONUS POSES:

1. YOGIC SQUAT

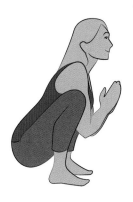

a. Stand in Mountain Pose.

b. Bend your knees, coming into a squatted position. Your knees should be out to the sides.

c. Place your upper arms inside your knees, bend them and place your palms together in Prayer Position.

d. Press your arms against your knees to open your squat. Keep your spine straight and your shoulders relaxed.

e. Take 5 deep breaths.

d. Return to Mountain Pose.

2. CHAIR TWIST

a. From Mountain Pose, bend your knees as if you are sitting in a chair.

b. Reach your arms up, then bring them into Prayer Position at the center of your chest.

c. Twist to the right and rest your left elbow on your right knee.

d. Take 5 deep breaths.

e. Stand.

f. Do the same on the opposite side.

g. Take 5 deep breaths.

h. Stand and return to Mountain Pose.

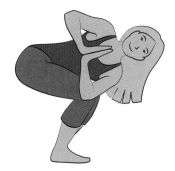

As I mentioned, Wall Street personalities often have jobs that require long days behind a desk, but our bodies were not made to sit on a chair for hours. Prolonged sitting is one of the major causes of sciatica. In addition to the 14-minutes of Wall Street Yoga every day, **stand from your desk at least once per hour.** Walk around. Gently stretch your body. *Breathe.* If possible, get some fresh air. Let go of your tension. Let go of your stress.

Bounce back like a rubber band.

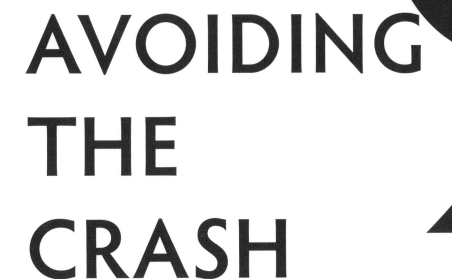

AVOIDING THE CRASH

Heart-healthy Yoga

"Disease is dis-ease. Yoga focuses on making your life *easier* by making your attitude easier."

- GuruNanda

A STOCK MARKET CRASH IS A SUDDEN, STEEP DECLINE

in stock prices, resulting in a significant financial loss. While Wall Street "suits" deal with a crash in the physical trenches, Wall Street *personalities* are confronted with a symbolic crash when health declines due to way of life. Ironically, economic crashes are driven by **panic** just like personal crashes. A personal crash can come in the physical form of diabetes and heart disease.

MY CRASH:

It was a regular office day. I was sitting at my desk. I had just slogged through horrendous traffic, during which time my wife and I had an argument on the phone over something trivial and dumb. I soon discovered that a huge shipment was delayed and that the delay could result in heavy penalties. I then opened a letter to learn that a former employee had filed a complaint that was completely false. Then came the news that my favorite salesman had decided to quit and join a competing company.

After years and years of this same cycle, it was just too much.

I started to have difficulty breathing. I opened the button on my pants, thinking maybe I had over-eaten (I had, but that's besides the point). My assistant came in with my morning coffee, but before my first sip, I felt piercing chest pain. Like a fish out of water, I gulped for air.

After a 9-1-1 call, I found myself at the hospital hooked up to an ECG machine. The doctor asked about my family history - my dad suffered two heart attacks and had several stents. He had diabetes since age 36. I was 38.

The doctor revealed that the ECG didn't look great. Given my family history, he talked of a possible angioplasty, going as far as to have my chest shaved for the procedure! "You may be going through cardiac arrest," he told me. I thought about an uncle who had undergone angioplasty and subsequently found out that he didn't need it! Medicine and lifestyle change would have resolved his heart issues. As a prolific reader, I was aware that angioplasty is overused.

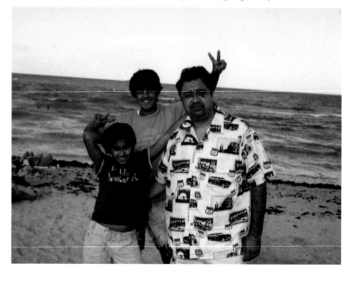

Ultimately, since my ECG did not deteriorate and tests came up negative, I did not need surgery. Instead, the doctor told me that I had suffered a severe anxiety attack, but that if I didn't make changes in my life, the next time could be much, much worse. Crash could mean "crash cart" for me.

That day was my real awakening.

Diabetes is a gateway to heart disease. It can also cause nerve, kidney, eye and foot damage, in addition to increasing the risk of osteoporosis, Alzheimer's Disease and certain cancers.

Diabetes and heart disease both evolve from a deadly combination of stress, unhealthy eating habits and lack of exercise.

A yogic way of life can help keep diabetes (i.e. high blood sugar levels) under control by:

- Reducing the glucagon secretions created by stress.
- Promoting weight loss.
- Relaxing muscles and improving blood circulation to the muscles. This action may enhance insulin glucose uptake, which reduces blood sugar.
- Lowering blood pressure. High blood pressure can instigate diabetes and related complications.
- Taming stress hormones like adrenaline, noradrenalin and cortisol.

This means that change is not only good. It's *lifesaving*. A study by the National Academy of Sciences reveals that a simple regimen of exercise, yoga and meditation actually "turns on" good, disease-preventing genes. It may even **slow the effects of aging** by increasing the amount of telomerase, an enzyme that affects cell growth. Similarly, research from American Heart Association demonstrates that yoga improves heart health in both fit individuals *and* those with diagnosed heart disease.

When it comes to *recovering* from surgery and medical procedures, studies have shown that the more yoga and meditation participants did, the more they improved. Many heart bypass patients experience depression, facing emotions ranging from anxiety to grief. In addition to physical recovery, yoga helps post-surgery patients with emotional recovery.

DON'T FORGET TO CONSULT A MEDICAL PROFESSIONAL before starting any kind of fitness program, including mine. There are caveats for those who have heart conditions. Know yours and adhere to them.

START THIS ROUTINE IN A SEATED, CROSS-LEGGED POSITION WITH YOUR SPINE STRAIGHT.

1. KAPALABHATI BREATHING

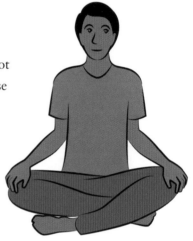

a. In your cross-legged position, rest your hands on your knees.

b. Through your *nose only*, take a deep breath and exhale quickly, making a "puff out" sound.

c. Focus on a forceful exhale, not on the inhale. Your chest will rise with every exhale.

d. Perform 20 breaths.

2. ALTERNATE NOSTRIL BREATHING

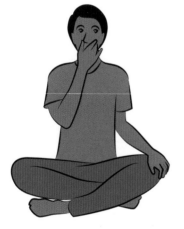

a. For this exercise, you will also breathe through your *nose only*. With your right thumb, close off your right nostril. Inhale through your left nostril.

b. Change to close off the left nostril with your right forefinger and exhale through your right nostril. Inhale through that right nostril.

c. Change to close off the right nostril with your right thumb and exhale through your left nostril. Inhale through that left nostril.

d. Change to close off the left nostril with your right forefinger and exhale through the right nostril. Your inhales should be through the same nostril, exhales through the opposite nostril.

c. Do each round 5 times.

3. BEE'S BREATH

a. Place your thumbs on the cartilage between your cheek and ear - the little flap that mutes your hearing when you press on it (not *in* your ear). Your elbows will be out to the side.

b. Put your other fingers over your eyes with your elbows out to the sides.

c. Take a deep breath and hum out a "bee buzzing" sound with your mouth closed. The sound should come from the bottom of your throat.

d. Focus on the center of your forehead to open up your "Third Eye" and feel the buzzing vibration inside your entire head.

e. Let out all your breath, then breathe in through your nose.

f. Do this 5 times.

g. Breathe and relax with your eyes closed. Feel the calming "buzzing" sensation radiate through your body and mind.

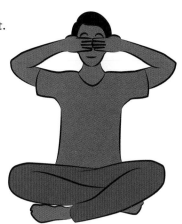

4. PALM TREE POSE

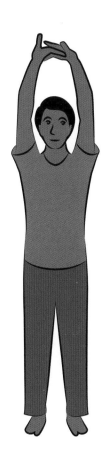

a. Stand tall in Mountain Pose with your feet parallel, hip distance apart. Lift your arms in the air.

b. Interlock your fingers and turn your hands so your palms face upward.

c. Lift your heels. Focus on a fixed object in front of you to maintain your balance.

d. Feel the pull upwards while your toes press into the floor. Remember to keep your shoulders relaxed - don't hunch them up by your ears.

e. Take 5 deep breaths all the way down to your navel.

f. Gently lower your heels, release your arms to your sides, and stand in Mountain Pose.

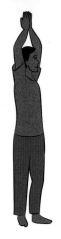

5. TWISTED TREE POSE

a. With your arms in the air, palms touching, twist at the waist to your right.

b. Take 5 deep breaths.

c. Twist to the left.

d. Take 5 deep breaths.

6. TRIANGLE POSE

a. Step your feet wide apart. Make sure that your hips are facing forward.

b. Turn your right leg, including your thigh, knee, and foot, out 90 degrees.

c. Turn your left leg in about 15 degrees.

d. Raise your arms to shoulder level, straight out, with your palms facing down. Inhale and stretch your upper body over your right leg.

e. Exhale and place your right hand on your right shin. Keep your chest open.

f. Raise your left arm toward the sky, with your palm facing forward. Gaze at your hand.

g. Take 5 deep breaths.

h. Return to standing.

i. Pivot your feet and do the other side.

j. Take 5 deep breaths.

k. Return to Mountain Pose.

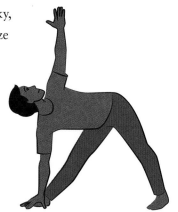

7. CAT-COW POSE

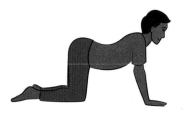

a. On your hands and knees, lift your belly button toward your spine to make your back flat. Your neck should be long and the top of your head forward.

b. Simultaneously, lift your head up and your bottom up, curving your back in a slight "U" shape.

c. Take 5 deep breaths.

d. Round your spine in an upside-down "U" shape.

e. Drop your head and gaze at your navel.

f. Take 5 deep breaths.

g. Do each pose once more.

h. Come back to neutral position with your back flat and the top of your head forward.

8. WESTERN'S POSE

• Sit with your legs straight out in front of you.

• Reach out and touch your toes. If you feel inflexible at first, bend your knees slightly.

• Take 10 deep breaths.

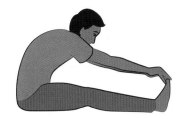

9. ONE-LEGGED SEATED TWIST

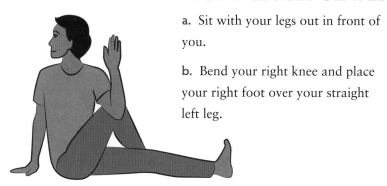

a. Sit with your legs out in front of you.

b. Bend your right knee and place your right foot over your straight left leg.

c. Place your elbow on the inside of your bent right leg. Your palm is in a "wave" position. Press your elbow against your knee so you can feel the twist in your waist.

d. Take 5 deep breaths.

e. Switch sides.

f. Take 5 deep breaths.

10. COBRA POSE

a. Lie on your stomach with your toes pointed.

b. Place your hands underneath your chest, palms down.

c. Press down to lift your torso up. Gaze up.

d. Take 5 deep breaths.

e. Release your torso down and relax.

f. Repeat once more.

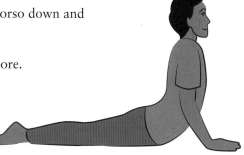

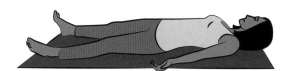

CORPSE POSE

BONUS POSES:

1. BRIDGE POSE

a. Lie on your back with your knees bent, feet on the floor, hip distance apart.

b. Lift up onto your toes.

c. Support your lower back with your hands and lift your bottom up. Your shoulders will remain touching the floor.

d. Take 5 deep breaths.

e. Gently lower your bottom to the floor.

2. PLOW POSE

a. Lie flat on your back.

b. Move your legs upward until they make a right angle with your upper body.

c. Support your lower back with your hands and lift your bottom up. Your shoulders will remain touching the floor.

d. Bring your legs over your head until your feet touch the floor past your head. Try and keep your legs straight.

e. Bring your arms away from your back toward the floor, palms down.

f. Take 5 deep breaths.

g. Roll your body carefully down until you're lying flat.

Diabetes and heart disease *are* genetic. But if we have knowledge of that physical constitution, we can take the steps necessary to avoid "crashing" like our parents or grandparents did. Yoga is a combination of the most meaningful steps:

MOVEMENT. BREATH. PEACE OF MIND.

Yoga enables us to put our healthiest foot forward and walk a path of well-being and longevity.

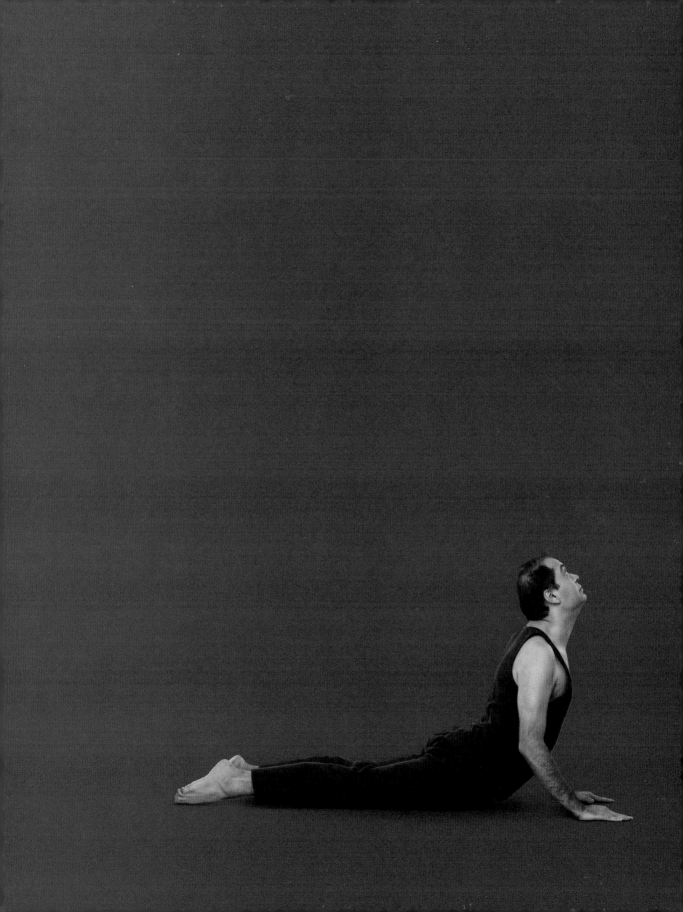

STEER YOUR 10 INVESTMENT

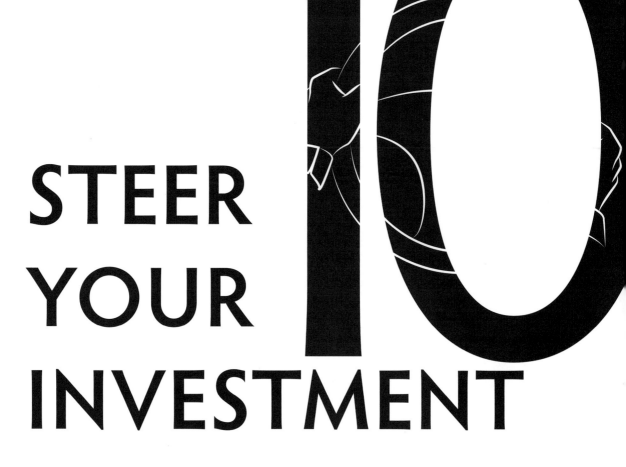

Yoga for Driving

"You're not stuck in traffic. You're released from the race for a moment."

- GuruNanda

MOST OF US SPEND A SIGNIFICANT AMOUNT OF TIME IN OUR CARS.

Data shows that during the past ten years, surface road miles increased only 1.1 percent while total miles traveled has increased 40 percent. That adds up to *more traffic*. If you're a businessperson, you're racing to the office. If you're a parent, you're trying to get your kids to school or activities on time. Often, we are both.

I live in Los Angeles, one of the most congested cities in the world. In my business, I drove all over the city, spending a majority of my time sitting in gridlock. When you are seated and strapped into your seatbelt behind the wheel of your car, your diaphragm is compressed. Breath cannot flow properly and your circulation is impaired.

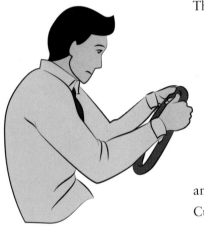

The longer you sit, especially in aggravating traffic, the more you risk:

- High blood pressure
- Elevated anxiety
- Headaches
- Constipation
- Stiff and sore muscles

If I wasn't in gridlock, I was constantly being confronted with angry, aggressive drivers. In the AAA Foundation's 2008 Traffic Safety Culture Index, 78% of respondents considered aggressive drivers serious safety threats. And with good reason. The National Highway Traffic Safety Administration estimates that approximately 33% of all motor vehicle accidents are due to aggressive driving.

Aggressive driving includes the following behaviors:

- Yelling
- Making angry, insulting or obscene gestures
- Cutting in front of other drivers
- Using the shoulder or a no-passing zone to pass
- Honking
- Flashing headlights

What if 100% of drivers LAUGHED instead? Not sarcastically, but with relief and good intentions.

Road Rage:

There have been countless times when I have been cut off or flipped off on the road. Even after doing yoga for so long, I can feel my insides start to rumble with anger. That kind of aggression aimed at us presses a universal hot button. We can choose to react like a firecracker bursting. The firecracker sets off a vicious cycle of unhealthy energy, negative hormones, and constricted blood circulation and breath. Or we can respond like the ocean that languidly flows over jagged rocks.

For me, the minute I let out one "Ho-ho-ha-ha-ha!" the anger dissolves. What could be better than to just laugh at the situation? I can't make the traffic go away, but I can make my stress *about it* go away. By laughing, *you* can transform the toxic energy that causes a stiff neck and muscle spasms into positive oxytocin that will calm your whole body.

You depend on the sturdiness and reliability of your car. The same should be true for your body. Driving is just one of the daily things you do that can cause stress. By practicing Wall Street Yoga and meditating everyday, you are preparing your body, mind and spirit for anything that comes along the road. Just 14 minutes a day will make whatever time you spend in your car easier and more enjoyable.

10 YOGIC DRIVING TIPS

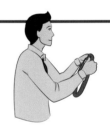

1. Sit tall, lifting up from the top of your head. By giving yourself maximum height, you can see better when you change lanes.
2. Hold the steering wheel with your hands at 3 and 9 o'clock, instead of 10 and 2. This is the new recommendation that will protect your hands if your airbag deploys.

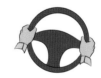

3. Avoid a "death grip" on the wheel. Are your knuckles white? Are your shoulders hunched up by your ears? Relax your arms, hands, shoulders, face and neck. Balance your focus and driving effort with relaxation.
4. Don't text and drive!
5. Avoid phone calls, especially those that may be upsetting.

6. Keep arguments or passionate discussions out of the car.
7. Listen to music that inspires good feelings. If rock music agitates you, try jazz or classical in your car.
8. Use stoplights as a moment to take an extra deep breath.

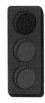

9. Make sure you keep easy breath flowing at all times.
10. Employ laughter yoga whenever necessary (and even when it's not).

Make efficient use of time and gain health by doing the following yogic breathing exercises during your daily commute. These will not only improve your mood, regardless of road conditions, they will counteract the diaphragm compression that occurs when sitting for long periods of time. And these simple moves can help save you from both health and road disasters.

"STEER YOUR INVESTMENT" ROUTINE

REMEMBER: *Keep your eyes wide open and your attention on the road, but still be aware of your breath.*

1. UJJAYI "VICTORY" BREATH

a. Inhale and exhale from the throat, through the *nose only*. A "hissing" sound should come from the upper part of the throat, not the nose.

b. Breathe in and out, slowly for 9 rounds. In your mind, count to 5 with each breath.

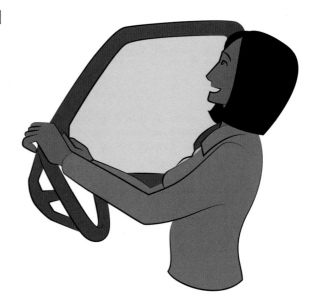

2. KAPALABHATI BREATHING

a. Through your *nose only*, take a deep breath and exhale quickly and sharply, making a "puff out" sound.

b. Focus on a forceful exhale, not on the inhale. Your chest will rise with every exhale.

c. Perform 20 breaths.

3. "OM" CHANT

Calm your mind by filling your head with the sound's vibration.

a. Take a deep breath in through your nose and release into "Om." Try and draw the sound out for as long as possible.

b. Do 3 long chants.

4. DRIVING LAUGHTER YOGA

The minute gridlock, honking and nasty drivers start to make you blow a gasket, laugh the negativity away. These chants can be done in any combination for as long as you feel you need them.

a. "Ha-ha-ha-ha-ha-ha-ha! Ha-ha-ha-ha-ha-ha-ha!"

b. "Very good! Very good! Very good!"

c. "Ho-ho-ha-ha-ha! Ho-ho-ha-ha! Ho-ho-ha-ha-ha! Ho-ho-ha-ha-ha!"

d. Breathe and calm down.

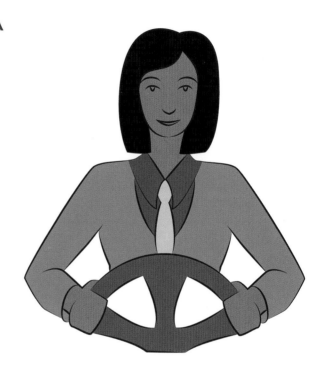

5. SLOW RELEASE BREATH

a. Through your *nose only*, very slowly inhale once, counting to 5 in your mind.

b. Exhale once through your *nose only,* counting to 6 in your mind.

If you don't have heart problems or blood pressure issues, you can count up to 10.

c. Repeat the cycle 3 times.

BONUS POSE:

If you *really* feel like you're exploding, pull over in a safe place - at the curb on a quiet street or in a parking lot. Turn off your motor and do this helpful breathing exercise.

ALTERNATE NOSTRIL BREATHING

Balance the right and left hemispheres of the brain, reducing anxiety.

a. For this exercise, you will also breathe through your *nose only*. With your right thumb, close off your right nostril. Inhale through your left nostril.

b. Change to close off the left nostril with your right forefinger and exhale through your right nostril. Inhale through that right nostril.

c. Change to close off the right nostril with your right thumb and exhale through your left nostril. Inhale through that left nostril.

d. Change to close off the left nostril with your right forefinger and exhale through the right nostril. Your inhales should be through the same nostril, exhales through the opposite nostril.

e. Do each round 5 times.

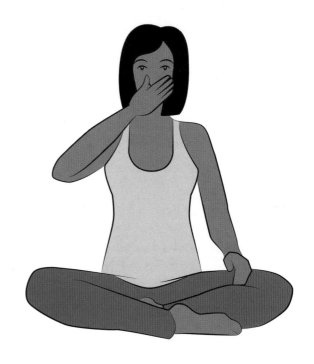

Remember, YOU are your most important investment. Steer that investment safely and calmly. You will get where you need to go. More importantly, *be* where you *are*, even if it's in the car.

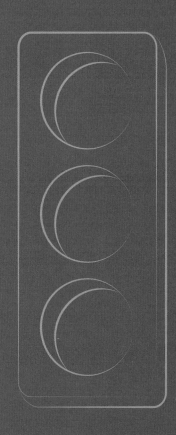

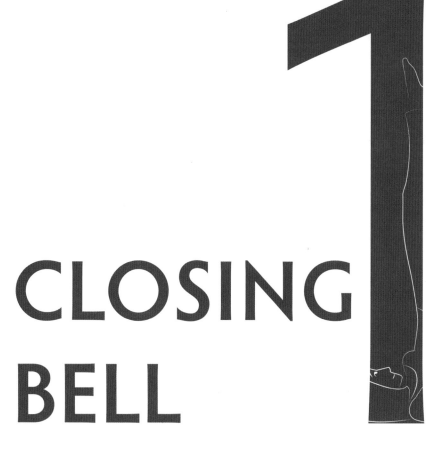

CLOSING
BELL

Yoga for Insomnia and Sleep Difficulties

"Sleep is the gift we give ourselves. Learn to unwrap yourself from your day."

- GuruNanda

WHETHER THE STOCK MARKET IS UP OR HAS TAKEN A TURN FOR THE WORSE, EACH DAY ENDS THE SAME WAY: Data with the ringing of the closing bell. As I mentioned, I have been lucky enough to ring the NYSE bell. At that time, I also was *unlucky* enough to suffer from insomnia. After regular 16-hour days, I would settle into bed only to be saddled with questions, struggles and general mind-chaos about my business, finances, family, schedules, travel... What had I accomplished? What *would* I accomplish? Was it enough? Would it ever be enough? I felt like I was riding a tiger, not running a business. If I tried to get off, the tiger would eat me. And when I kept riding, each part of my body cried out in exhaustion. There was always more, more, more to do - and none of that included a sound sleep. Needless to say, the next day would be filled with yawns and extra trips for double espressos.

Wall Street personalities sleep less because they never feel finished with work. This is not just the businessman or woman, but the stay-at-home mom who is organizing family schedules or helping a child go through challenging times like social drama or college applications. Or it might be today's overwhelmed student with an endless amount of homework and assignments. A Wall Street personality may go to bed on time - or even early - but life's demands keep him or her awake in bed, tossing and turning.

Insomnia, also known as sleeplessness, is a sleep disorder from which you, too, suffer if you:
1. Have difficulty falling asleep.
2. Experience trouble staying asleep.
3. Inadvertently and consistently wake up too early in the morning.
4. Feel tired when you get up.

Insomnia can cause of the following health issues:
* Depression
* Low immunity
* High blood pressure
* Heart disease
* Diabetes
* Memory loss

You and I are not alone, although it might feel that way in the middle of the night when everyone else is enjoying peaceful zzz's while your eyes are wide open and your mind is racing. Between 50 million and 70 million Americans suffer from sleep disorders or sleep deprivation, according to a 2009 report from the Centers for Disease Control (CDC).

> ## Adults typically need seven to eight hours of sleep a night.

When you're sick with a cold or flu, you feel sleepier, right? That's because Mother Nature needs to do her job and heal you during slumber. Sleep is crucial to our well-being all the way around.

Consequently, sleeping pill use has skyrocketed. Approximately 13 million Americans use sleeping pills, as estimated by the National Center for Health Statistics.

I, personally, couldn't fall asleep without the help of a prescribed sleep aid… until I integrated yoga and meditation into my nightly routine. People who practice yoga do everything consciously and with intention. That includes sleep. Flopping into bed fully awake and just expecting to fall asleep is actually laziness. You need to give your sleep process the care and time you would anything else that's important in your life. How *much* time? 14 MINUTES (including your 2 minutes of meditation twice a day). That's **JUST 14 EXTRA MINUTES A DAY FOR SEVERAL HOURS OF INCREDIBLE SLEEP.**

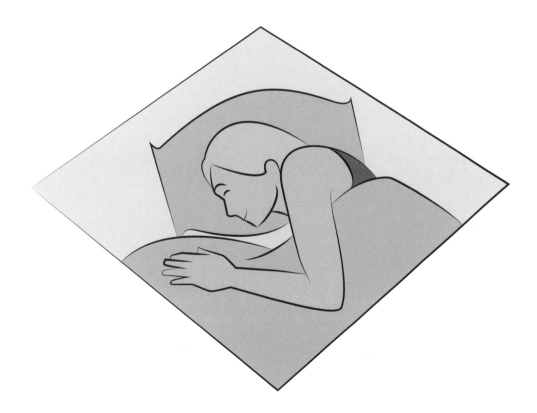

SET YOUR SIGHTS ON A RESTFUL SLEEP IN THE EARLY EVENING.

Then, follow these **BEDTIME DON'T'S**:

- **DON'T** drink caffeinated beverages, like coffee and soda. If you must drink tea, make it an herbal variety, like chamomile or mint.
- **DON'T** drink alcohol, which throws your sleep patterns out of whack. N-REM sleep (also know as "deep sleep") increases, incrementally decreasing REM (or "Rapid Eye Movement" rest/dream sleep). A *balance* of both is key, and alcohol disrupts this balance.
- **DON'T** play video games or watch television, especially action shows or movies.
- **DON'T** exercise rigorously in the evening. For some people, working out later rather than earlier can be a sleep "thief" because exercise releases adrenaline. Gentle yoga is a calming early evening alternative.

Getting ready for bed doesn't just mean brushing your teeth (though given my background as Dr. Fresh, I'm a big proponent of good oral care). Your bedtime routine should include these **DO'S**:

- A half-hour prior to sleep, **DO** drink tepid water to quench any thirst.
- **DO** something relaxing, like reading, knitting or Sudoku. Save the exciting or emotional books for daytime reading. At night, pick up something mindless or even boring.
- **DO** turn off your cellphone, laptop and tablet. The "blue light" from these electronics is thought to suppress your body's sleep-producing melatonin. I used to check my phone when I got up at 2 or 3 in the morning to see if I had any messages. That light took over and so did my struggle with sleep.
- **DO** create a peaceful bedroom environment:
- Close the door and dim the lights.
- Make sure your bedroom is dark and quiet.
- Adjust the room temperature to moderate - not too hot, not too cold.
- **DO** quell the "inside traffic" - the noise outside means less if you are quiet *inside*.

"CLOSING BELL" ROUTINE

I don't claim that yoga can put insomnia completely to bed, but it has helped me and many others manage the frustrating issue without the need for drugs. **FOR THE BEST RESULTS, THIS ROUTINE SHOULD BE DONE 3-4 HOURS BEFORE BEDTIME AND A HALF-HOUR BEFORE DINNER.** You will usher in your entire night by resting your body, mind and spirit, and avoid amping up too much before bed.

Sit in a cross-legged seated position on a mat or blanket. Start with your 2-minute mantra-based meditation, which is covered in Chapter 4. This is the close parentheses to your day.

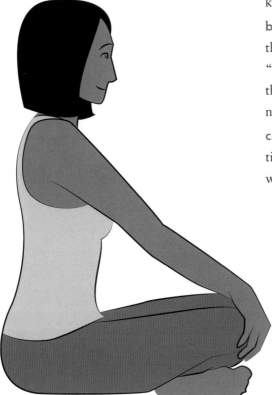

1. UJJAYI "VICTORY" BREATH

a. Remain in the cross-legged seated position with your spine straight. Rest your hands on your knees.

b. Inhale and exhale from the throat, through the *nose only*. A "hissing" sound should come from the upper part of the throat, not the nose.

c. Breathe in and out, slowly, 10 times. In your mind, count to 5 with each breath.

2. BEE'S BREATH

a. Sitting tall, place your thumbs on the cartilage between your cheek and ear - the little flap that mutes your hearing when you press on it (not *in* your ear).

b. Put your other fingers over your eyes with your elbows out to the sides.

c. Take a deep breath and hum out a "bee buzzing" sound with your mouth closed. The sound should come from the bottom of your throat.

d. Focus on the center of your forehead to open up your "Third Eye" and feel the buzzing vibration inside your entire head.

e. Let out all your breath, then breathe in through your nose.

f. Do this 5 times.

g. Breathe and relax with your eyes closed. Feel the calming "buzzing" sensation radiate through your body and mind.

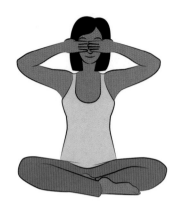

3. FORWARD FOLD POSE

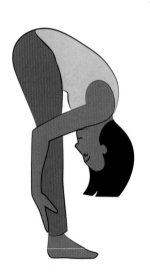

a. Stand proud in Mountain Pose with your feet parallel, hip distance apart. Inhale and reach your arms up.

b. Exhale as you slowly fold your upper body from the hips and try to touch your toes. If you feel inflexible, bend your knees slightly. You'll experience a gentle stretch in your hamstrings.

c. Let your head, upper body and hands hang loosely.

d. Take 10 deep breaths. With every exhale, try and touch your fingers to your toes.

e. Roll your body up one vertebrae at a time and stand in Mountain Pose.

4. CHILD'S POSE

a. Sit on your knees and reach your arms out in front of you, folding your torso over your thighs. Keep your bottom down.

b. With flat palms, spread your fingers wide. Your face should be close to the floor.

c. Take 5 deep breaths.

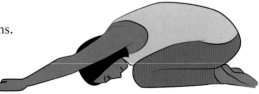

5. DOWNWARD-FACING DOG POSE

a. Start on your hands and knees.

b. Push down on your hands and lift your bottom up to the sky, straightening your arms and legs. You will be in an inverted "V" position.

c. Take 5 deep breaths.

d. Go back to your hands and knees.

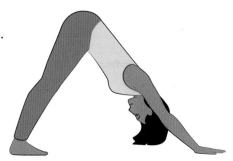

6. WESTERN'S POSE

a. Sit with your legs straight out in front of you.

c. Reach out and touch your toes. If you feel inflexible at first, bend your knees slightly.

d. Take 10 deep breaths.

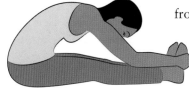

7. BRIDGE POSE

a. Lie on your back with your knees bent, feet on the floor, hip distance apart.

b. Lift up onto your toes.

c. Support your lower back with your hands and lift your bottom up. Your shoulders will remain touching the floor.

d. Take 5 deep breaths.

e. Gently lower your bottom to the floor.

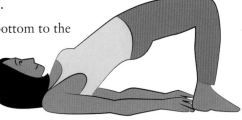

8. FISH POSE

This is the most important pose at the end of your day. It opens your chest and heart, inviting you to take in oxygen more fully.

a. Remain on your back with your legs long and straight. Place your hands underneath your bottom, palms down.

b. Lift up on your elbows.

c. Tilt your head back, so the top of your head touches the floor.

d. Flex your feet and press your heels away from you.

e. Take 5 deep breaths.

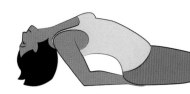

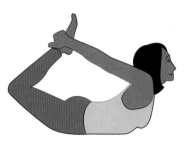

9. BOW POSE

a. Lie on your stomach.

b. Flex your feet and bend your knees.

c. Lift your feet up and reach back for them with your hands.

d. Holding your ankles, lift your legs. If you can't reach your ankles at first, just reach your arms back and your legs up.

e. Take 5 deep breaths.

10. HAPPY BABY POSE

a. Lie on your back.

b. Bend your knees to your chest.

c. Flex your feet.

d. Grab your feet with your hands and gently pull down so your knees are pressed toward the outside of your body. You will emulate the look of a cute, happy baby.

e. Rock slightly right and left

f. Take 5 deep breaths.

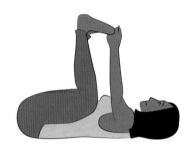

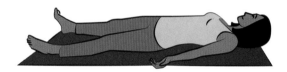

CORPSE POSE

BONUS POSES:

1. ALTERNATE NOSTRIL BREATHING

a. Sit in a cross-legged position. For this exercise, you will breathe through your *nose only.* With your right thumb, close off your right nostril. Inhale through your left nostril.

b. Change to close off the left nostril with your right forefinger and exhale through your right nostril. Inhale through that right nostril.

c. Change to close off the right nostril with your right thumb and exhale through your left nostril. Inhale through that left nostril.

d. Change to close off the left nostril with your right forefinger and exhale through the right nostril. Your inhales should be through the same nostril, exhales through the opposite nostril.

e. Do each round 5 times.

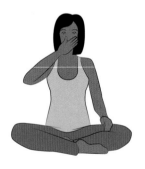

2. SHOULDER STAND

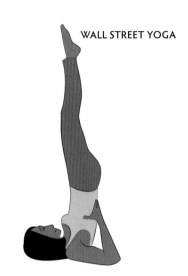

a. Lie on your back. Bend your knees and lift your feet off the floor.

b. Support your lower back with your hands.

c. As you lift your legs up toward the ceiling, your bottom will raise as well.

d. Straighten your legs and point your toes to the sky. You will be resting on your shoulders.

e. Take 5 deep breaths.

f. Slowly roll back down until you are lying flat. Release your arms.

With these moves, **your breath is the Number One component.** If you breathe and relax, you will organically help slow down your heart rate and calm your nervous system. The day's toxins will virtually release from your body and your cells will "open and free." These are not just physical toxins, but psychological ones. Negative thoughts will drift away, replaced by positive energy and affirmations. This action relieves your overall stress and anxiety, and promotes a deep and consistent sense of calm and confidence.

Since these yoga asanas don't take much time, you will see that they will quickly become a welcome part of your nighttime routine, just like washing your face and brushing your teeth.

If you do the Closing Bell Routine and find that you're still tossing and turning, then don't fight it! Get up and "finish" whatever is on your mind. Write down your thoughts. If you're upset with someone, compose an email, but *don't* send it. Use it to get out the feelings that are plaguing your sleep. Tossing and turning is a vicious cycle, actually *creating* anxiety. And don't look at the clock - that makes it worse.

Now, let's address sleep apnea. Sleep apnea is caused by a blockage of the airway, when the soft tissue in the back of the throat relaxes too much during slumber and virtually collapses down. It is akin to very severe, loud snoring. The body has a natural urge to breathe and you wake up, gasping for air. You're neither sleeping nor breathing. The cycle of apnea repeats over and over again throughout the night, making it impossible to get a restful sleep. The main cause of sleep apnea? Excess weight. I was a sleep apnea sufferer before I started practicing yoga and eating healthily. After I lost 40 pounds, the sleep apnea stopped. Studies show that losing as little as 14 pounds causes dramatic improvement. A weight loss of 40 pounds or more revealed a 58% reduction in sleep apnea symptoms.

Lastly, love your work - whether it's an office job, a traveling sales position, a creative career, parenting, or studying. If you're excited to wake up in the morning and forge ahead into your day, make sleep *consciously constructive.*

I say, **BETTER SLEEP, BETTER LIFE.**

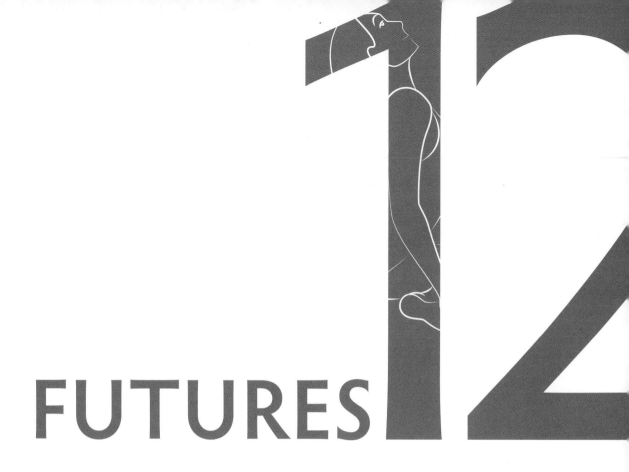

FUTURES12

Beyond Wall Street Yoga

"Love, connection and community are better than the best prescription drugs."

- GuruNanda

ON WALL STREET, A FUTURES CONTRACT IS AN EXCHANGE-TRADED

contract that requires delivery of a commodity, bond, currency or stock index, on a specific future date. It's basically a pledge. When you commit to yoga and meditation, you are pledging to deliver PRANA to yourself. Except there is no future date.

THE TIME IS NOW.

REMEMBER YOUR B.O.N.D.

BREATH - Yoga asanas (poses) and yogic breathing allow for an uninterrupted flow of oxygen and nutrients.

OPTIMISM - Positive thinking builds on itself. The more you see the glass as half full, the more you will have to drink because your attitude will lead you to approach life that way.

NUTRITION - Eating foods in their most natural, organic state and *in moderation* gives your body exactly what it needs.

DEEDS - Right action and generosity create good karmic energy. Simply, what goes around comes around.

Loosely wrap *yourself* around the EIGHT "LIMBS" OF YOGA and the foundation of well-being will grow inside you. Yoga isn't just about the poses. It's about breathing the movements to connect your body, mind and spirit. PRANA. LIFE FORCE.

Enjoy the P.U.R.E. System:

PERSPIRATION

URINATION

RESPIRATION

EXCRETION

I will always be a Wall Street personality, and I'm proud of my business successes. I will forever invent new products and formulas. That entrepreneurial spirit is in my DNA. But I've learned that there is so much more to life than productivity and profits.

When it comes to yoga, drop the expectations and do not seek results. I promise they will come. This attitude will infuse your entire existence. As Bhagavad Gita said, "It is better to live your own life imperfectly than to live an imitation of someone else's life with perfection."

All you need is consistency. **14 MINUTES A DAY.** Consistency is the magic trick. Your body is the wand.

INTERACT. Participating in positive social interactions with the people you love releases that "cuddle hormone." Your body, mind and spirit will grow and strengthen. Negative interaction will do the opposite. **THE CHOICE IS YOURS.**

Transform the Maelstrom of Misery into a Sea of Serenity. When you balance yourself through a yogic lifestyle, everyone else benefits. Your healthy energy flows outward and softly bathes the people around you.

SEA OF SERENITY

THE WORLD

⬆

SIGNIFICANT OTHER

⬆

THE WORLD ⬅ FRIENDS ⬅ YOU ➡ KIDS ➡ THE WORLD

⬇

COLLEAGUES

⬇

THE WORLD

In upcoming GURUNANDA'S HAPPY BREATH YOGA books, I will explore more ways of dealing with our world - efficiently, yet profoundly. Subjects will include:

- Diet, nutrition and weight loss
- Relationships and intimacy
- Parenting
- Growing up
- Mid-life
- Traveling
- And more

Please visit me at WWW.GURUNANDA.COM to find out about new developments:

- Online yoga pose instructional videos
- Happy Breath Yoga breathing seminars
- Private mantra-creation sessions
- DVD sets
- Apps
- Products and tools (like neti pots and pulling oils)

I want to make life easier for you. More importantly, I want you to learn to *make life easier for yourself.*

The stock market is volatile. For investors, this can be unnerving and stressful. You're either worried about an investment you should have bought in the past or concerned about how one will perform in the future. But the smartest financial minds believe that the market always steadies... like life.

Be healthy. Breathe. But better, BREATHE HAPPY.

NAMASTE.

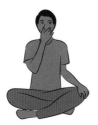

ALTERNATE NOSTRIL BREATHING

1. Sit in a cross-legged position. You can also do this exercise in a chair or in your car (if you are parked with the motor off).

2. For this exercise, you will breathe through your nose only. With your right thumb, close off your right nostril. Inhale through your left nostril.

3. Change to close off the left nostril with your right forefinger and exhale through your right nostril. Inhale through that right nostril.

4. Change to close off the right nostril with your right thumb and exhale through your left nostril. Inhale through that left nostril.

5. Change to close off the left nostril with your right forefinger and exhale through the right nostril. Your inhales should be through the same nostril, exhales through the opposite nostril.

6. Do each round 5 times.

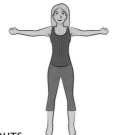

ARM-OUTS

1. Start in Mountain Pose.

2. Lift your arms straight out to the side and make tight fists. Circle your arms 20 times clockwise, then 20 times counter-clockwise.

3. Keep your arms straight out and flex your wrists up and down 20 times.

4. Keep your arms straight out and circle your hands at the wrist. Do 10 circles each direction.

5. Bring your arms back down and stand in Mountain Pose.

Balancing Tree Pose

1. Stand in Mountain Pose.

2. Balance on the right leg and bend the left leg, turning the left knee out.

3. Place the sole of the left foot on the right calf or thigh. (Do not place the sole of the foot on the knee. This can produce a knee injury).

4. Balance with your arms down or in the air. If your arms are in the air, you can place your palms together with your fingers pointed up.

5. Focus your eyes on one point to help you balance.

6. Take 5 deep breaths.

7. Do the opposite side.

8. Return to Mountain Pose with your hands in Prayer Position and take 1 deep breath.

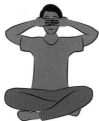

BEE'S BREATH

1. Sit in a cross-legged position, keeping your spine straight. You can also do this exercise in a chair.

2. Place your thumbs on the cartilage between your cheek and ear - the little flap that mutes your hearing when you press on it (not in your ear). Your elbows will be out to the side.

3. Put your other fingers over your eyes.

4. Take a deep breath and hum out a "bee buzzing" sound with your mouth closed. The sound should come from the bottom of your throat.

5. Focus on the center of your forehead to open up your "Third Eye" and feel the buzzing vibration inside your entire head.

6. Let out all your breath, then breathe in through your nose.

7. Do this 5 times.

8. Breathe and relax with your eyes closed. Feel the calming "buzzing" sensation radiate through your body and mind.

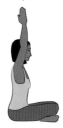

BELLOW'S BREATH

If you have high blood pressure, do this exercise with your arms relaxed on your thighs. Breathe gently.

1. Sit in a cross-legged position, spine straight. You can also do this exercise in a chair.

2. Press your arms up with a swift inhale through your nose only.

3. Pull your arms down with a swift exhale through your nose only.

4. Your chest will puff out when you inhale, retract when you exhale.

5. Repeat 10 times.
6. Relax your arms and take a deep breath.

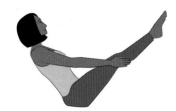

BOAT POSE

1. Sit with your knees bent.
2. Keep your abs firm and lift your legs.
3. Straighten your legs.
4. Reach your arms past your knees. If you need help balancing, lightly hold on to your thighs.
5. Take 5 deep breaths.
6. Bend your knees and put your feet back on the floor.
7. Lay back and relax.

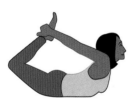

BOW POSE

1. Lie on your stomach.
2. Flex your feet and bend your knees.
3. Lift your feet up and reach back for them with your hands.
4. Holding your ankles, lift your legs. If you can't reach your ankles at first, just reach your arms back and your legs up.
5. Take 5 deep breaths.

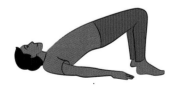

BRIDGE POSE

1. Lie on your back with your knees bent, feet on the floor, hips' distance

apart.
2. Lift up onto your toes.
3. Support your lower back with your hands and lift your bottom up. Your shoulders will remain touching the floor.
4. Take 5 deep breaths.
5. Gently lower your bottom to the floor.

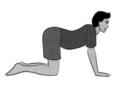
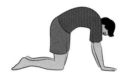

CAT-COW POSE

1. On your hands and knees, lift your belly button gently toward your spine to make your back flat. Your neck should be long and the top of your head forward.
2. Simultaneously, lift your head up and your bottom up, curving your back in a slight "U" shape.
3. Take 5 deep breaths.
4. Round your spine in an upside-down "U" shape.
5. Drop your head and gaze at your navel.
6. Take 5 deep breaths.
7. Do each pose once more.
8. Come back to neutral position with your back flat and the top of your head forward.

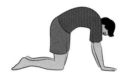

CHAIR POSE

1. Start in Mountain Pose.
2. Inhale and raise your arms straight up next to your ears.

3. Exhale and bend your knees as if you are sitting in a chair. Try and get your thighs parallel to the floor with your bottom pushed out.
4. Lift your heart as you breathe, bringing your hips even lower (though never below your knees). Keep your arms straight up. If you need "training wheels," hold onto the back of a chair for balance.
5. Take 5 deep breaths.
6. Inhale with a higher lift of the arms and stand in Mountain Pose, bringing your arms down.

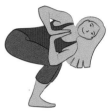

CHAIR TWIST

1. Start in Mountain Pose.
2. Bend your knees as if you are sitting in a chair.
3. Reach your arms up, then bring them into Prayer Position at the center of your chest.
4. Twist to the right and rest your left elbow on your right knee.
5. Take 5 deep breaths.
6. Stand.
7. Do the same on the opposite side.
8. Take 5 deep breaths.
9. Stand and return to Mountain Pose.

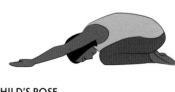

CHILD'S POSE

1. Sit on your knees and reach your arms out in front of you, folding your torso over your thighs. Keep your bottom down.
2. With flat palms, spread your fingers wide. Your face should be close to the floor.
3. Take 5 deep breaths.

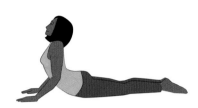

COBRA POSE

1. Lie on your stomach with your toes pointed.
2. Place your hands underneath your chest, palms down.
3. Press down to lift your torso up. Gaze up.
4. Take 5 deep breaths.
5. Release your torso down and relax.
6. Repeat once more.

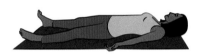

CORPSE "SHAVASANA" POSE

1. Lie on your back. Your feet should be hips' distance apart and your arms are by your sides. Your palms are facing up.
2. Close your eyes.
3. Take 3 deep breaths through your nose only.
4. Start progressively relaxing - from your toes up to your shins… knees… thighs… hips… stomach… chest… arms… neck… and forehead. You will finally feel like your entire body is heavy and melted into the floor. Your breath will become shallow - that's okay.
5. Pretend that you are looking at your body from above. Be in that awareness state for ONE MINUTE - you are a spectator, not your body itself.
6. Gently roll onto your right side and slowly sit up.

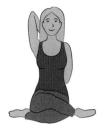

COW'S FACE POSE

1. Sit with both legs straight out.
2. Bend your right leg in front of you, knee and calf flat on the floor.
3. Lift your left leg, bend your knee and place your left knee on top of your right knee. Your left calf should be stacked horizontally on top of your right calf. If someone were looking at you, your legs would look like a cow's mouth!
4. Reach your right arm up and your left arm down.
5. Reach them behind you and try to clasp your hands. Don't worry if your hands don't reach each other. Just go for the stretch in your shoulders and across your chest.
6. Take 5 deep breaths.
7. Do the same thing with the other leg and the opposite arm position.
8. Take 5 deep breaths.

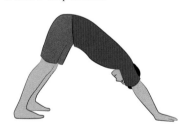

DOWNWARD-FACING DOG POSE

1. Start on your hands and knees.
2. Push down on your hands and lift your bottom up to the sky, straightening your arms and legs. You will be in an inverted "V" position.
3. Take 5 deep breaths.
4. Go back to your hands and knees.

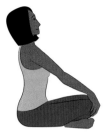

FIRE'S BREATH

1. Sit in a cross-legged position. You can also do this exercise in a chair or in your car - anywhere you can keep your back straight.
2. As you take a deep breath in for 5 counts through your nose only, feel it deep in your stomach. Simultaneously, pull your stomach up toward the ribs, so it will look hollowed out.
3. Exhale through your nose and release your stomach.
4. Repeat once more.

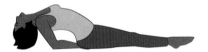

FISH POSE

1. Lie on your back with your hands underneath your bottom, palms down.
2. Lift up on your elbows.
3. Tilt your head back, so the top of your head touches the floor.
4. Flex your feet and press your heels away from you.
5. Take 5 deep breaths.

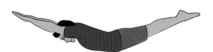

FLYING POSE

1. Lie on your stomach.
2. Reach your arms out in front of your head.
3. Keep your legs straight and point your toes.
4. Lift your arms and legs. You might not

get far off the ground.
5. Take 5 deep breaths.

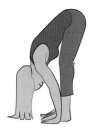

FORWARD FOLD POSE

1. Stand in Mountain Pose. Inhale, reaching up.
2. Exhale as you slowly fold your upper body from the hips and try to touch your toes. If you feel inflexible, bend your knees slightly. You'll experience a gentle stretch in your hamstrings.
3. Let your head, upper body and hands hang loosely.
4. Take 10 deep breaths. With every exhale, try and touch your fingers to your toes.
5. Roll your body up one vertebrae at a time and stand in Mountain Pose.

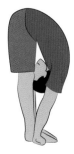

FORWARD FOLD WITH FISTS

1. From Mountain Pose, fold forward.
2. Try to keep your legs straight. If you feel inflexible, bend your knees slightly.
3. Bend your elbows out to the sides, laying one forearm on top of the other.
4. Make fists and squeeze them.
5. Take 10 deep breaths.
6. Release your hands and arms and let them hang to the floor.
7. Roll up with a round back and stand in Mountain Pose.

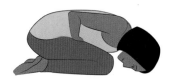

FROG POSE
(TRADITIONAL INDIAN VERSION)

1. Sit on your knees.
2. Make fists and bring them together so that your thumbs touch your navel. Your elbows will be out to the sides.
3. Exhale and lean forward over your fists. Try to touch your chest to your knees.
4. Take 5 deep breaths.
5. Sit up and relax.
6. Repeat once more.

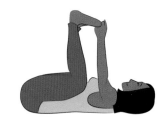

HAPPY BABY POSE

1. Lie on your back.
2. Bend your knees to your chest.
3. Flex your feet.
4. Grab your feet with your hands and gently pull down so your knees are pressed toward the outside of your body. You will emulate the look of a cute, happy baby.
5. Rock slightly right and left.
6. Take 5 deep breaths.

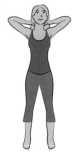

HEAD PRESS

1. Stand in Mountain Pose. Put your hands behind your head with your palms facing you.
2. Press your head back against your hands. Keep your head straight.
3. Take 5 deep breaths.
4. Press your right palm against the right side of your head. Keep your head straight.
5. Take 5 deep breaths.
6. Press the left palm against the left side of your head. Keep your head straight.
7. Take 5 deep breaths.
8. Press both palms against your forehead. Keep your head straight.
9. Take 5 deep breaths.

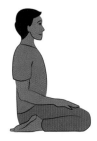

HERO'S POSE

1. Sit on your knees.
2. Put your palms on your thighs.
3. When you become more flexible, you can slide your bottom to the floor.
4. Take 5 deep breaths.

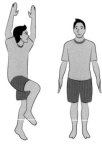

THE JACKPOT

1. Standing, throw your arms up and let your body burst with victory as if you've just won the lottery!
2. Laugh "Haaaa! Haaaa!" as you pump your arms, kick your legs, shake your bottom - whatever feels good.
3. Continue for 30 seconds.
4. Stand tall in Mountain Pose.
5. Breathe and calm down.

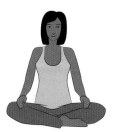

KAPALABHATI BREATHING

1. Sit in a cross-legged position. You can also do this exercise in a chair or in your car - anywhere you can keep your back straight.
2. Through your nose only, take in a deep breath and exhale quickly and sharply, making a "puff out" sound.
3. Focus on a forceful exhale, not on the inhale. Your chest will rise with every exhale.
4. Perform 20 breaths.

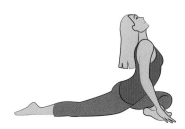

KING PIGEON POSE

1. Start on your hands and knees.
2. Slide your right knee forward toward your left hand and lay it down so your knee is facing out. Your foot should be underneath your chest.
3. Press your palms into the floor and your arms straight. Your chest should be forward, along with your head.
4. Take 5 deep breaths.
5. Move back to your hands and knees.
6. Do the other side.
7. Take 5 deep breaths.

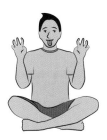

THE LION

1. Sit in a cross-legged position on the floor. You can also do this exercise seated in a chair. Make "claws" with your hands.
2. Roar like a lion as you move across your body like you are scaring predators. Repeat across your body 2 more times.
3. Throw your arms in the air in celebration as you say "Ha-ha-ha-ha-ha!" Repeat 2 more times.
4. Put your thumbs and forefingers together by your sides and say "Very good! Very good!" as you move right, then left.
5. Say "Very good!" 1 time toward the middle.
6. Clap your hands as you chant "Ho-ho-ha-ha-ha!" The "ho-ho" is to your left, the "ha-ha-ha" to your right. Repeat 2 more times.
7. Rest your hands on your knees.
8. Breathe and calm down.
Note: You can also do this exercise silently.

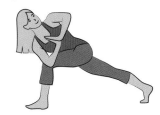

LUNGE TWIST

1. From Mountain Pose, lunge forward with your right foot.
2. Put your palms together in Prayer Position, elbows out to the side.
3. Twist your upper body to the right and place your left elbow on your right knee.
4. Take 5 deep breaths.
5. Repeat on the left side.

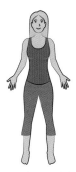

MOUNTAIN POSE

1. Stand tall with your spine straight and your head proud.
2. Place your feet parallel, hips' distance apart.
3. Let your arms hang loosely by your sides.
4. Breathe deeply.

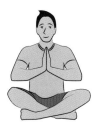

THE NAMASTE

1. Sit on the floor in a cross-legged position, with your palms together in Prayer Position at the center of your chest. You can also do this exercise in a chair.
2. Quickly repeat "Ha-ha-ha-ha-ha-ha-ha!" while moving your upper body across your lower body, right to left then left to right. Repeat 2 more times in both directions.
3. Throw your arms in the air in celebration as you say "Ha-ha-ha-ha-ha!" Repeat 2 more times.
4. Put your thumbs and forefingers together by your sides and say "Very good. Very good!" as you move right, then left.
5. Say "Very good!" 1 time toward the middle.
6. Clap your hands to the chant "Ho-ho-ha-ha-ha!" The "ho-ho" is to your left, the "ha-ha-ha" to your right. Repeat 2 more times.
7. Rest your hands on your knees.

8. Breathe and calm down.

Note: You can also do this exercise silently.

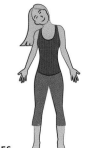

NECK STRETCHES

1. Stand in Mountain Pose.
2. Bend your head to the right, then the left. Do this slowly with 1 deep breath for each side.
3. Repeat 5 times each side. Every time, you should be able to take your head further.

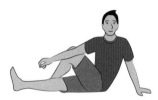

ONE-LEGGED SEATED TWIST

1. Sit with your legs out in front of you.
2. Bend your right knee and place your right foot over your straight left leg.
3. Place your elbow on the inside of your bent right leg. Your palm is in a "wave" position. Press your elbow against your knee so you can feel the twist in your waist.
4. Take 5 deep breaths.
5. Switch sides.
6. Take 5 deep breaths.

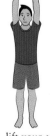

PALM TREE POSE

1. From Mountain Pose, lift your arms in the air.
2. Interlock your fingers and turn your hands so your palms face upward.

3. Lift your heels. Focus on a fixed object in front of you to maintain your balance.
4. Feel the pull upwards while your toes press into floor. Remember to keep your shoulders relaxed - don't hunch them up by your ears.
5. Take 5 deep breaths all the way down to your navel.
6. Gently lower your heels, release your arms to your sides and stand in Mountain Pose.

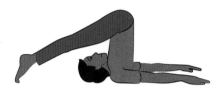

PLOW POSE

1. Lie flat on your back.
2. Move your legs upward until they make a right angle with your upper body.
3. Support your lower back with your hands and lift your bottom up. Your shoulders will remain touching the floor.
4. Bring your legs over your head until your feet touch the floor past your head. Try and keep your legs straight.
5. Bring your arms away from your back toward the floor, palms down.
6. Take 5 deep breaths.
7. Roll your body carefully down until you're lying flat.

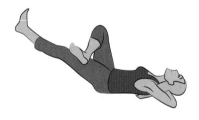

RECLINED THIGH OVER THIGH POSE

1. Lie on your back with your legs bent. Put your hands behind your head, elbows out.
2. Cross your right leg over your left.
3. Twist your lower body toward the left.

Try and get your crossed legs to touch the floor.
4. Take 5 deep breaths.
5. Cross your left leg over your right.
6. Twist your lower body toward the right.
7. Take 5 deep breaths.

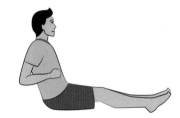

THE ROWING

1. Sit on the floor in a cross-legged position. You can also do this exercise in a chair. Pretend you are holding an oar with both hands.
2. Row 1 time to the right while saying "Ha!" then once to the left while saying "Ha!" Repeat 4 more times both sides, rowing faster and faster.
3. Throw your arms in the air in celebration as you say "Ha-ha-ha-ha-ha!" Repeat 2 more times.
4. Put your thumbs and forefingers together by your sides and say "Very good! Very good!" as you move right, then left.
5. Say "Very good!" 1 time toward the middle.
6. Clap your hands as you chant "Ho-ho-ha-ha-ha!" The "ho-ho" is to your left, the "ha-ha-ha" to your right. Repeat 2 more times.
7. Rest your hands on your knees.
8. Breathe and calm down.

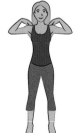

SHOULDER ROLLS

1. Stand in Mountain Pose.
2. Bend your arms and bring your hands to

your shoulders.

3. Make full, slow circle rotations, keeping your fingers at your shoulders. These circles should be as big as possible. Do 10 forward.

4. Do 10 backwards.

5. Return to Mountain Pose.

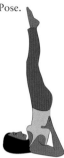

SHOULDER STAND

1. Lie on your back. Bend your knees and lift your feet off the floor.

2. Support your lower back with your hands.

3. As you lift your legs up toward the ceiling, your bottom will raise as well.

4. Straighten your legs and point your toes to the sky. You will be resting on your shoulders.

5. Take 5 deep breaths.

6. Slowly roll back down until you are lying flat. Release your arms.

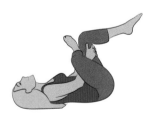

SIMPLIFIED PIGEON POSE

1. Lie on your back with your knees bent.

2. Turn your right knee out and put your right foot on your left knee.

3. Wrap your hands around your left thigh and gently put your legs toward you.

4. Take 5 deep breaths.

5. Do the same on the opposite side.

6. Take 5 deep breaths.

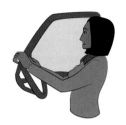

SLOW RELEASE BREATH

1. Sit on the floor in a cross-legged position. You can also do this exercise in a chair or in your car.

2. Through your nose only, very slowly inhale once, counting to 5 in your mind.

3. Exhale once through your nose only, counting to 6 in your mind. If you don't have heart problems or blood pressure issues, you can count up to 10.

4. Repeat the cycle 3 times.

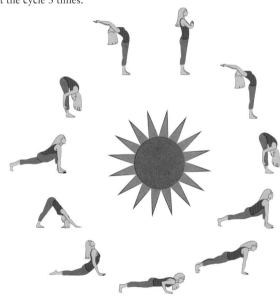

SUN SALUTATION

A simple rule for breathing during this exercise: breathe out as you move graciously toward Mother Earth, breath in as your raise yourself to stand tall against the pressures of life. This "in and out" is important for balancing ego, work, and life in general.

1. Stand in Mountain Pose with your palms together in Prayer Position, thumbs touching your heart.

2. Inhale and reach your arms up and slightly back. Gaze toward the sky, feeling a long stretch from neck to feet.

3. Exhale and fold forward from your hips. Touch your hands to the floor. Bend your knees slightly if you feel inflexible.

4. With your hands on the floor, inhale and extend your right leg back in a lunge. You can put your knee down or keep it lifted.

5. Bring your left foot back and exhale, lowering your knees and calves to the floor.

6. With an inhale, press your palms into the floor and straighten your arms to push your torso up in Cobra Pose.

7. Exhale, lifting your bottom to the sky and straightening your legs in Downward-Facing Dog Pose.

8. Inhale and bring your right foot forward, back into a lunge.

9. Exhale and bring your left foot to meet your right in a Forward Fold.

10. Inhale and roll your upper body up to standing.

11. Exhale in Mountain Pose, hands to Prayer Position.

For 10 Sun Salutations, do 5 with the right leg first, then 5 with the left.

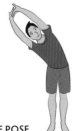

SWAYING PALM TREE POSE

1. Standing in Mountain Pose, interlock your fingers with your index fingers pointed up, and raise your arms.

2. Ground yourself into the floor while distributing weight equally between your feet.

3. Keep your hips forward and bend at the waist to your right. Take 5 deep breaths. Feel the stretch on the side of your torso, but don't let your hips lose their straight alignment.

4. Bend at the waist to your left and take 5 deep breaths.

5. Do the right and left side again, extending a little further with each exhalation.

6. Return to Mountain Pose.

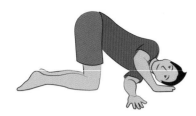

THREAD THE NEEDLE POSE

1. On your hands and knees, slide the right hand underneath your body and across your chest to the left.

2. Your right shoulder and side of the head should sit comfortably on the floor.

3. Take 5 deep breaths.

4. Switch arms.

5. Take 5 deep breaths.

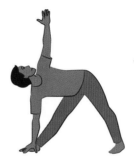

TRIANGLE POSE

1. From Mountain Pose, step your feet wide apart. Make sure that your hips are facing forward.

2. Turn your right leg, including your thigh, knee and foot, out 90 degrees.

3. Turn your left leg in about 15 degrees.

4. Raise your arms to shoulder level straight out, with your palms facing down. Inhale and stretch your upper body over your right leg.

5. Exhale as you place your right hand on your right shin. Keep your chest open.

6. Raise your left arm toward the sky, with your palm facing forward. Gaze at your hand.

7. Take 5 deep breaths.

8. Return to standing.

9. Pivot your feet and do the other side.

10. Take 5 deep breaths.

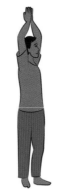

TWISTED TREE POSE

1. Stand in Mountain Pose.

2. Lift your arms in the air and press your palms together.

3. Twist at the waist to your right.

4. Take 5 deep breaths.

5. Twist to the left.

6. Take 5 deep breaths.

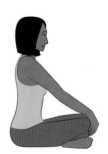

UJJAYI "VICTORY" BREATH

1. Sit on the floor in a cross-legged position. You can also do this exercise in a chair or in your car.

2. Through your nose only, inhale and exhale from the throat. A "hissing" sound should come from the upper part of the throat, not the nose.

3. Breathe in and out, slowly for 9 rounds. In your mind, count to 5 with each breath.

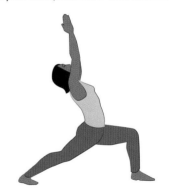

WARRIOR 1 POSE

1. Stand tall in Mountain Pose, then step your feet wide apart.

2. With your hands on your hips, turn your right leg and foot out 90 degrees while you turn your left leg and foot in 45 degrees.

3. Square your chest in the direction of your right leg.

4. Inhale and lift your arms above your head. Bring your palms together.

5. Exhale and bend your right knee to a 90-degree angle.

6. Take 5 deep breaths.

7. Straighten your right leg and return to Mountain Pose.

8. Repeat on the other side.

9. Take 5 deep breaths.

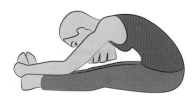

WESTERN'S POSE

1. Sit with your legs straight out in front of you.
2. Reach out and touch your toes. If you feel inflexible at first, bend your knees slightly.
3. Take 10 deep breaths.

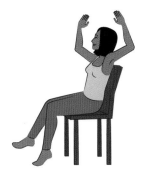

WILD GIBBERISH

1. Start on the floor in a cross-legged position. You can also do this exercise in a chair.
2. Let yourself go wild with sounds, words and grunts that don't make any sense. Talk, sing, cry, shout, mumble, whisper! Express whatever needs to be expressed and throw everything out!
3. Allow your arms and body to lose control with your sounds to totally release your energy. Flop over, flap, kick, punch!
4. Do this for 30 seconds without stopping.
5. Rest your hands on your knees.
6. Breathe and calm down. In the stillness and silence, feel how the catharsis - the "letting go" - has penetrated your whole body, from head to toe.

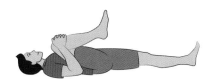

WIND REMOVING POSE

1. Lie on your back.
2. Pull your right leg into your chest, bent.
3. Take 5 deep breaths.
4. Release the leg back to the floor, straight.
5. Pull your left leg into your chest, bent.
6. Take 5 deep breaths.

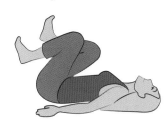

YOGIC CYCLING - BENT LEGS

1. Lying on your back, bend your knees with your feet lifted. Your calves should be parallel to the floor.
2. Slowly cycle your legs. Make sure you keep your core tight, pulling your belly button toward the floor. This will ensure your back stays down flat.
3. Cycle 20 times, both legs.

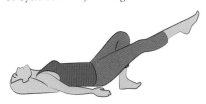

YOGIC CYCLING - STRAIGHT LEGS.

1. Lying on your back, lift your right leg to a 45-degree angle. Keep it straight, with only a slight bend at the knee, and point your toes.
2. Circle your leg 10 times one direction, then 10 times the other direction.

3. Do the same cycling with the left leg at a 45-degree angle. Remember to keep your core tight and your back flat.

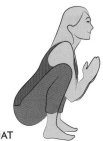

YOGIC SQUAT

1. Stand in Mountain Pose.
2. Bend your knees, coming into a squatted position. Your knees are out to the sides.
3. Place your upper arms inside your knees, bend them and place your palms together in Prayer Position.
4. Press your arms against your knees to open your squat. Keep your spine straight and your shoulders relaxed.
5. Take 5 deep breaths.
6. Return to Mountain Pose.

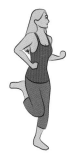

YOGIC JOGGING

1. Jog in place using both legs. Bring your knees up as high as you comfortably can. Circle your arms gently by your sides. Do 50 jogs.
2. Do 50 more jogs, kicking your feet toward your bottom. Remember to try and control your breath. Don't pant. Instead, breathe.
3. Rest in Mountain Pose.

REFERENCES

"Aggressive Driving Enforcement: Strategies for Implementing Best Practices" (1998) National Highway Traffic Safety Administration.

"Aggressive Driving Research Update." (2009) AAA Foundation for Traffic Safety.

Aljasir, B., Bryson, M., and Al-shehri, B. "Yoga Practice for the Management of Type II Diabetes Mellutus in Adults: A systematic review." *Evidence-Based Complementary and Alternative Medicine.* Dec 2010; 7(4): 399-40.

Cahn, B. and Polich, J. "Meditation States and Traits: EEG, ERP, and Neuroimaging Studies." *Psychology of Consciousness: Theory, Research, and Practice* 1.S (2013): 48-96.

Chong, Y., Fryar, C., and Gu, Q. "Prescription Sleep Aid Use Among Adults: United States, 2005–2010". *National Center for Health Statistics.* Issue brief no. 12. 2013.

Deffenbacher, J.L., Deffenbacher, D.M., Lynch, R.S., & Richards, T.L. "Anger, aggression and risky behavior: A comparison of high and low anger drivers." *Behaviour Research and Therapy* (2003) 41(6), 701-718.

Deffenbacher, J.L., Filetti, L.B., Richards, T.L., Lynch, R.S., & Oetting, E.R. "Characteristics of two groups of angry drivers." *Journal of Counseling Psychology* (2003) 50(2), 123-132.

Friedman, M., & Rosenman, R. H. "Association of specific overt behavior pattern with blood and cardiovascular findings." *Journal of the American Medical Association* (1959) 169, 1286-1296.

Gonzalez, O., Berry, J., McKnight-Eily, L., Strine, T., Edwards, V., Lu, H. et al. "Current Depression Among Adults - United States, 2006 and 2008" *Morbidity and Mortality Weekly Report* (2010) 59(38);1229-1235.

Hoy, D., March, L., Brooks, P., Blyth, F., Woolf, A. & Bain, C., et al. "The global burden of low back pain: estimates from the Global Burden of Disease 2010 study" *Annals of Rheumatic Diseases/The Eular Journal* (2014) 73:6 968-974.

Johansson, K., Hemmingsson, E., Harlid, R., Lagerros, Y., Granath, F., Rossner, S., et al. "Longer term effects of very low energy diet on obstructive sleep apnoea in cohort derived from randomised controlled trial: prospective observational follow-up study" *BMJ* 2011;342:d3017.

Luders, E., Kurth, F., Mayer, E., Toga, A., Narr, K., & Gaser, C. "The unique brain anatomy of meditation practitioners: alterations in cortical gyrification" (2012) *Frontiers in Human Neuroscience.*

Manocha, R., Gordon, A., Black, D., Malhi, G. Seidler, R. "Using Meditation for Less Stress and Better Wellbeing: A Seminar for GP's" (2009) *Australian Family Physician.* Volume 30, No. 6.; 454-8.

Martin, R. "Humor, laughter, and physical health: methodological issues and research findings." *Psychological Bulletin.* 2001 Jul;127(4):504-19.

Moadel, A., Shah, C., Wylie-Rosett J, et al. "Randomized controlled trial of yoga among a multiethnic sample of breast cancer patients: effects on quality of life." (2007) *Journal of Clinical Oncology*. 2007;25:4387-4395.

"National Survey of Speeding and Unsafe Driving Attitudes and Behaviors" (2003) National Highway Traffic Safety Administration (NHTSA).

Ornish, D., Magbanua, M., Weidner, G., Weinberg, V., Kemp, Coleen, Green, C., et al. "Changes in prostate gene expression in men undergoing an intensive nutrition and lifestyle intervention." (2008) *Proceedings of the National Academy of Sciences of the United States of America.*

"Prescription Drug Abuse and Overdose. Public Health Perspective." (2012) Centers for Disease Control and Prevention.

Raghavendra, M., Nageendra, H., Raghuram, N., Vinay, C., Chandrashekara, S., Gopinath, K., et al. "Influence of yoga on postoperative outcomes and wound healing in early operable breast cancer patients undergoing surgery." *International Journal of Yoga*. 2008 Jan-Jun; 1(1): 33–41.

"Relieving Pain in America: A Blueprint for Transforming Prevention, Care, Education, and Research." (2011) Institute of Medicine. Washington, DC: The National Academies Press.

Schrank, D., Eisele, B., & Lomax, T. *T.T.I's 2012 Urban Mobility Report*. (2012) Texas A&M Transportation Institute. The Texax A&M University System.

Sivasankaran, S. "The Effect of a Six-Week Yoga Training and Meditation Program on Endothelial Function." (2004). American Heart Association Scientific Sessions.

"Sleep Disorders and Sleep Deprivation: An Unmet Public Health Problem." (2006). Institute of Medicine. Washington, DC: The National Academies Press.

Soni, A. "Back Problems: Use and Expenditures for the U.S. Adult Populations, 2007." *Statistical Brief #289. Medical Expenditure Panel Survey*. (2010) Agency for Healthcare Research and Quality.

"Traffic Safety Culture Index." (2009) AAA Foundation for Traffic Safety.

"Unhealthy Sleep-Related Behaviors - 12 States, 2009" *Centers for Disease Control and Prevention - Morbidity and Mortality Weekly Report* (2011) Vol. 60/No.

Note: This information may not cover all possible claims, uses, actions, precautions, side effects or interactions. It is not intended as medical advice, and should not be relied upon as a substitute for consultation with your doctor, who is familiar with your medical situation.

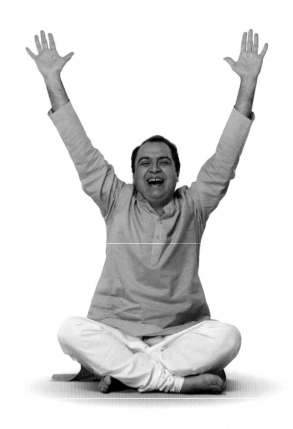